T0226652

Procedures in the Office Setting

Editors

TONY OGBURN
BETSY TAYLOR

OBSTETRICS AND GYNECOLOGY CLINICS OF NORTH AMERICA

www.obgyn.theclinics.com

Consulting Editor
WILLIAM F. RAYBURN

December 2013 • Volume 40 • Number 4

ELSEVIER

1600 John F. Kennedy Boulevard • Suite 1800 • Philadelphia, Pennsylvania, 19103-2899

http://www.theclinics.com

OBSTETRICS AND GYNECOLOGY CLINICS OF NORTH AMERICA Volume 40, Number 4
December 2013 ISSN 0889-8545, ISBN-13: 978-0-323-26112-8

Editor: Kerry Holland
Developmental Editor: Yonah Korngold

Obstetrics and Gynecology Clinics (ISSN 0889-8545) is published quarterly by Elsevier Inc., 360 Park Avenue South, New York, NY 10010-1710. Months of issue are March, June, September, and December. Periodicals postage paid at New York, NY, and additional mailing offices. Subscription price per year is $310.00 (US individuals), $545.00 (US institutions), $155.00 (US students), $370.00 (Canadian individuals), $688.00 (Canadian institutions), $255.00 (Canadian students), $450.00 (foreign individuals), $652.00 (foreign institutions), and $225.00 (foreign students). To receive student/resident rate, orders must be accompanied by name of affiliated institution, date of term, and the signature of program/residency coordinator on institution letterhead. Orders will be billed at individual rate until proof of status is received. Foreign air speed delivery is included in all *Clinics* subscription prices. All prices are subject to change without notice. POSTMASTER: Send address changes to *Obstetrics and Gynecology Clinics*, Elsevier Health Sciences Division, Subscription Customer Service, 3251 Riverport Lane, Maryland Heights, MO 63043. **Customer Service: Telephone: 1-800-654-2452 (U.S. and Canada); 314-447-8871 (outside U.S. and Canada). Fax: 314-447-8029. E-mail: journalscustomerservice-usa@elsevier.com (for print support); journalsonlinesupport-usa@elsevier.com (for online support).**

Reprints. For copies of 100 or more of articles in this publication, please contact the Commercial Reprints Department, Elsevier Inc., 360 Park Avenue South, New York, New York 10010-1710. Tel.: 212-633-3874; Fax: 212-633-3820; E-mail: reprints@elsevier.com.

Obstetrics and Gynecology Clinics of North America is also published in Spanish by McGraw-Hill Interamericana Editores S.A., P.O. Box 5-237, 06500, Mexico; in Portuguese by Reichmann and Affonso Editores, Rio de Janeiro, Brazil; and in Greek by Paschalidis Medical Publications, Athens, Greece.

Obstetrics and Gynecology Clinics of North America is covered in MEDLINE/PubMed (Index Medicus), Excerpta Medica, Current Concepts/Clinical Medicine, Science Citation Index, BIOSIS, CINAHL, and ISI/BIOMED.

Printed and bound by CPI Group (UK) Ltd, Croydon, CR0 4YY

Transferred to digital print 2012

Contributors

CONSULTING EDITOR

WILLIAM F. RAYBURN, MD, MBA
Chair, Department of Obstetrics and Gynecology; Associate Dean, Continuing Medical Education, University of New Mexico School of Medicine, Albuquerque, New Mexico

EDITORS

TONY OGBURN, MD
Professor, Department of Obstetrics and Gynecology, Chief Medical Officer, University of New Mexico Sandoval Regional Medical Center, University of New Mexico Health Sciences Center, Albuquerque, New Mexico

BETSY TAYLOR, MD
Assistant Professor and Chief, Division of General Obstetrics and Gynecology, Department of Obstetrics and Gynecology, University of New Mexico Health Sciences Center, Albuquerque, New Mexico

AUTHORS

REBECCA H. ALLEN, MD, MPH
Assistant Professor, Department of Obstetrics and Gynecology, Women and Infants Hospital, Warren Alpert Medical School of Brown University, Providence, Rhode Island

ANITRA BEASLEY, MD, MPH
Assistant Professor, Department of Obstetrics and Gynecology, Baylor College of Medicine, Houston, Texas

SAWEDA BRIGHT, MD
Chief Resident in Obstetrics and Gynecology, Virginia Commonwealth University Health System, Richmond, Virginia

DANIELLE COOPER, MD
Assistant Professor of Obstetrics and Gynecology, Associate Program Director, Louisiana State University Health Sciences Center, Shreveport, Louisiana

ALISON EDELMAN, MD, MPH
Associate Professor, Co-Director, Family Planning Fellowship, Department of Obstetrics and Gynecology, Oregon Health and Science University, Portland, Oregon

JONATHAN L. GLEASON, MD
Female Pelvic Medicine and Reconstructive Surgery, Assistant Professor of Obstetrics and Gynecology and Surgery, Virginia Tech Carilion School of Medicine, Carilion Clinic, Roanoke, Virginia

KELLY R. HODGES, MD
Assistant Professor, Division of Gynecologic and Obstetric Specialists, Department of Obstetrics and Gynecology, Baylor College of Medicine, Houston, Texas

JOHN P. KEATS, MD, CPE, FACOG, FACPE
Assistant Clinical Professor of Obstetrics and Gynecology, The David Geffen School of Medicine, University of California, Los Angeles, Los Angeles, California

LAWRENCE M. LEEMAN, MD, MPH
Professor, Department of Family and Community Medicine, University of New Mexico; Professor, Department of Obstetrics and Gynecology, University of New Mexico, Albuquerque, New Mexico

EDWARD J. MAYEAUX Jr, MD, DABFP, FAAFP
Professor and Chairman, Department of Family and Preventive Medicine; Professor of Obstetrics and Gynecology, University of South Carolina School of Medicine, Columbia, South Carolina

ELIZABETH MICKS, MD, MPH
Acting Assistant Professor, Department of Obstetrics and Gynecology, University of Washington, Seattle, Washington

JOHN G. PIERCE Jr, MD
Associate Professor of Obstetrics and Gynecology and Internal Medicine, Virginia Commonwealth University Health System, Richmond, Virginia

JORDAN PRITZKER, MD, MBA, FACOG
Womens Health and Wellness, Woodbury, New York

ANN SCHUTT-AINÉ, MD
Assistant Professor, Department of Obstetrics & Gynecology, Baylor College of Medicine, Houston, Texas

LAURIE S. SWAIM, MD
Director, Division of Gynecologic and Obstetric Specialists, Baylor College of Medicine; Chief, Gynecology, The Pavilion for Women, Texas Children's Hospital, Houston, Texas

BETSY TAYLOR, MD
Assistant Professor and Chief, Division of General Ob/Gyn, Department of Obstetrics and Gynecology, University of New Mexico Health Sciences Center, Albuquerque, New Mexico

SARAH WOODS, MD
Department of Obstetrics and Gynecology, University of Tennessee Health Science Center, Memphis, Tennessee

NICOLE YONKE, MD, MPH
Assistant Professor, Department of Family and Community Medicine, University of New Mexico, Albuquerque, New Mexico

Contents

OBSTETRICS AND GYNECOLOGY CLINICS

FORTHCOMING ISSUES

March 2014
Recurrent First Trimester Pregnancy Loss
William H. Kutteh, MD, PhD, *Editor*

June 2014
Addiction Disorders During Pregnancy
William F. Rayburn, MD, MBA, and
Hilary Smith Connery, MD, *Editors*

September 2014
Pelvic Pain
Mary T. McLennan, MD, *Editor*

RECENT ISSUES

September 2013
Breast Disorders
Victoria L. Green, MD, JD, MBA, and
Patrice M. Weiss, MD, *Editors*

June 2013
HPV, Colposcopy, and Prevention of Squamous Anogenital Tract Malignancy
Alan G. Waxman, MD, MPH, and
Maria Lina Diaz, MD, FACOG, *Editors*

March 2013
Obstetric Emergencies
James M. Alexander, MD, *Editor*

Foreword

Obstetric and Gynecologic Procedures in the Office

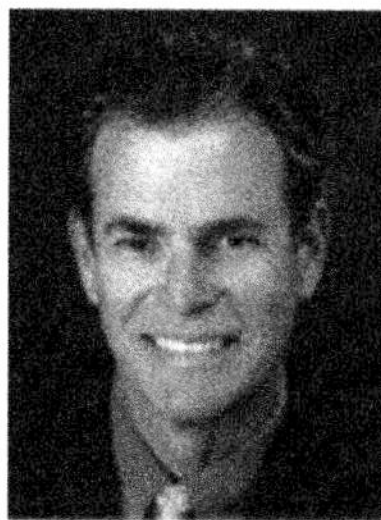

William F. Rayburn, MD, MBA
Consulting Editor

This issue of *Obstetrics and Gynecology Clinics of North America*, edited by Dr Tony Ogburn and Dr Betsy Taylor, identifies the best topics for discussion about procedures to be performed in the ambulatory or office setting. I believe that the material presented here by qualified authors will be of great interest to you in your office gynecology practice. Noninvasive procedures are being offered more as alternatives to surgery, as medical treatment becomes more dominant in today's clinical practice. In addition, indications for minimal-invasive surgery continue to expand.

Many procedures routinely performed by the obstetrician-gynecologist can be now performed efficiently in a less costly manner at a free-standing or hospital-based ambulatory surgical facility or office that offers more patient satisfaction. The office setting is one type of an ambulatory surgical facility. Examples of procedures that can often be performed safely in ambulatory settings include endometrial sampling, endometrial ablation, loop electrosurgical excision procedure, hysteroscopy for diagnostic or therapeutic reasons, follicular aspiration, long-term contraceptive insertions, surgical abortion, cystoscopy, and a variety of vulvar procedures.

In planning this edition, the guest editors recognized that management philosophies vary widely. An effort is made throughout the issue to consider practice styles and algorithms that highlight key management strategies. As mentioned in each section of the issue, office-based procedures should be limited to those that can be performed safely; are consistent with staff expertise and equipment; and are in accordance with the intrinsic risk of the procedure, the patient's condition, and satisfactory pain relief. Procedures performed in the office should be those for which there is a reasonable expectation of discharge within a short period with recovery occurring easily at home. A report on optimizing reimbursement with appropriate coding for office-based procedures has particular relevance.

Obstet Gynecol Clin N Am 40 (2013) ix–x
http://dx.doi.org/10.1016/j.ogc.2013.09.005
0889-8545/13/$ – see front matter

We should anticipate the number of office-based practices to grow in the ensuing decade with fewer hospitalizations being necessary beyond treatment of certain cancer or pelvic support disorders. I appreciate this contemporary overview about patient selection, resources needed, and helpful tips described by the authors. We look forward to a timely update in the next 10 years.

William F. Rayburn, MD, MBA
Chair, Department of Obstetrics and Gynecology
Associate Dean, Continuing Medical Education
University of New Mexico School of Medicine
MSC10 5580, 1 University of New Mexico
Albuquerque, NM 87131-0001, USA

E-mail address:
wrayburn@salud.unm.edu

Preface

Procedures in the Office Setting

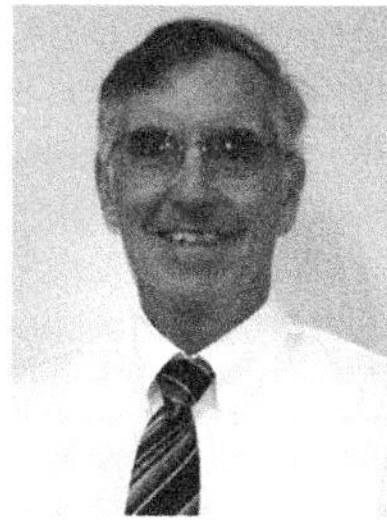
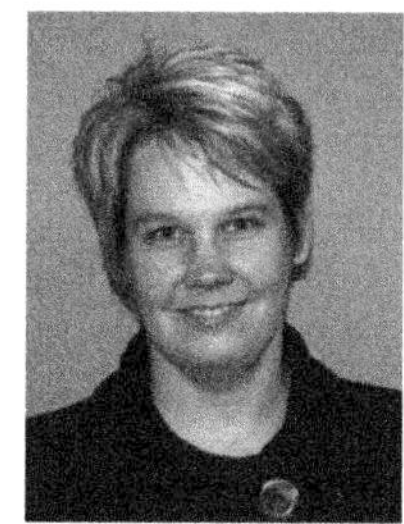

Tony Ogburn, MD Betsy Taylor, MD
Editors

The practice of Obstetrics and Gynecology has evolved tremendously in the past several decades to include an increasing emphasis on procedures performed in an office-based setting. Many procedures, once performed only in an operating room under anesthesia, are now routinely performed in the office. The reasons for this change are multifaceted. Patient convenience and satisfaction are important factors that have contributed to the shift to office procedures. Patients may feel more comfortable with the familiar surroundings of their doctor's office. Often parking, access, and the time commitment are more favorable in an office setting. From the provider perspective, performing the procedure in the office can be much less disruptive to the daily schedule as it eliminates the travel time between the hospital and the office and typically schedules in the office are more efficient than operating room schedules. For example, in the office setting other patients can be seen between cases, while in the OR this time is typically lost. Financial considerations also influence the shift to the office setting. The expenses associated with operating an inpatient facility are typically much greater than an office setting and the overall costs to the system for a procedure are often much higher in the operating room. It can be cost saving for the patient and payers to perform procedures in the office. Reimbursement to the provider may differ significantly between the office and inpatient or ambulatory surgery center.

Despite the advantages that exist to encourage performance of procedures in the office setting, providers must consider a number of issues before doing so. First and foremost is patient safety. The incidence of complications and the ability to manage them should be equivalent between the operating room and clinic. Patient satisfaction should be equivalent or better in the office setting but will depend on the availability of adequate pain control and support. Outcomes should be equivalent between the two settings. The ability to complete a procedure or obtain an adequate specimen should

Obstet Gynecol Clin N Am 40 (2013) xi–xiii
http://dx.doi.org/10.1016/j.ogc.2013.09.004 **obgyn.theclinics.com**
0889-8545/13/$ – see front matter

not be compromised. The necessary equipment, space, and trained support staff must be available, which may be more challenging in the office setting, especially if the volume of procedures performed is low. Finally, performing a procedure in the office with the patient awake and without the more extensive resources available in the operating room may challenge the provider's skills and comfort level. Adequate training and preparation for the provider and staff are essential.

In this issue of *Obstetrics and Gynecology Clinics of North America* we bring together a diverse group of outstanding authors to provide a resource for the provider performing or planning to perform procedures in the office setting. Several articles have widespread applicability to any provider. As noted above, patient safety and comfort are paramount to successful performance of office procedures. Dr John Keats provides a useful summary of the requirements for the office and how they can be implemented and used. Drs Allen, Micks, and Edelman review the most successful approaches to pain control available in the office setting and provide useful tips to optimize patient comfort. Dr Pritzker provides an excellent summary explaining the appropriate coding for office procedures and highlights the differences that exist between coding and billing in the office versus the operating room.

The remaining articles cover the most commonly performed office procedures in women's health. Each article provides a helpful review of patient selection, resources needed, and helpful tips for success in the office. Drs Leeman and Yonke review techniques of surgical abortion including management of spontaneous abortion as well as elective termination. They provide details on the use of the manual vacuum aspirator, an inexpensive but highly effective device that enables management of abortion to be done effectively in the office without the need for a much more expensive electronic suction machine. Drs Hodges and Swaim review hysteroscopic sterilization, a procedure rapidly gaining in popularity. They discuss the use of the hysteroscope in the office setting, which can be used for other indications in addition to sterilization. Drs Pierce and Bright discuss the range of procedures used to evaluate and treat cervical dysplasia, the vast majority of which are now performed in the office setting. Drs Taylor and Woods provide a useful review of the various types of global ablation techniques, which are an excellent alternative for many women for the management of abnormal bleeding. Dr Beasley and Schutt-Ainé provide a discussion of long-acting reversible contraceptives, including both implants and intrauterine devices. These methods provide the most effective contraception for most women but as they gain in popularity it is important for providers to know how to manage the occasional difficult insertion or removal. Drs Mayeaux Jr and Cooper cover an extensive array of vulvar procedures that can be performed in the office setting with a focus on selection of the optimal approach to each lesion. Finally Dr Gleason provides a review of cystoscopy, a diagnostic procedure often used in the workup of gynecologic conditions including incontinence.

In addition to the outstanding effort of the authors we would like to thank the editors and staff at Elsevier for their guidance and patience in the development of this issue. We hope women's health providers will find this a useful resource to assist them in providing safe, effective procedures in the office setting.

Tony Ogburn, MD
Department of Obstetrics and Gynecology
MSC 10 5580
1 University of New Mexico
Albuquerque, NM 87131, USA

Betsy Taylor, MD
Department of Obstetrics and Gynecology
MSC 10 5580
1 University of New Mexico
Albuquerque, NM 87131, USA

E-mail addresses:
jogburn@salud.unm.edu (T. Ogburn)
btaylor@salud.unm.edu (B. Taylor)

Patient Safety in the Obstetric and Gynecologic Office Setting

John P. Keats, MD, CPE

KEYWORDS

- Patient safety • Office safety • SCOPE program • Medical leadership
- Office policy and procedure manual • Checklists • Mock drills • Safety culture

KEY POINTS

- Many opportunities exist to reduce the risk of patient harm in the office setting.
- Appointing a medical director for patient safety in the office is an important first step.
- Establishing a culture whereby safety issues can be discussed openly is the foundation of safe office practice.
- Communication with patients in a way that is easily understood by them will improve safety.
- Medication safety is as important in the office setting as in the hospital.
- The use of checklists and mock drills will reduced the risk of adverse surgical events in the office procedure room.

INTRODUCTION

The modern era of the patient safety movement in the United States was ushered in by the Institute of Medicine's release in 1999 of *To Err is Human*[1] and in 2001 of its sister publication *Crossing the Quality Chasm*.[2] These publications served as a resounding wake-up call to the fact that patients were being harmed, and often killed, on a daily basis by medical errors in American hospitals. Many of these errors were and are preventable, and the years since have seen tremendous efforts made by hospitals and medical professional organizations to enhance awareness of patient safety issues. These initial efforts at improving patient safety were focused almost entirely on patient care rendered in the hospital setting. Despite these efforts, it is unclear how much progress has been made in reducing harm to patients that is attributable to medical errors.[3] However, the work done on patient safety improvement projects in the hospital have allowed the identification of the areas of greatest vulnerability that allow errors to reach patients in the form of adverse medical events. These "holes in the Swiss cheese," as per the model of adverse events proposed by James Reason,[4] have

Department of Obstetrics and Gynecology, The David Geffen School of Medicine, University of California, Los Angeles, 10833 Le Conte Avenue, Los Angeles, CA 90095, USA
E-mail address: JKeatsMD@gmail.com

Obstet Gynecol Clin N Am 40 (2013) 611–623
http://dx.doi.org/10.1016/j.ogc.2013.08.004 obgyn.theclinics.com
0889-8545/13/$ – see front matter

become the subject of scrutiny and endeavors to devise ways to close these safety gaps and thus intercept errors before harm ensues.[5] These strategies appear to have equal applicability in the office or outpatient setting, although only more recently has it been realized that risks to patient safety exist in these areas as well.[6]

RISKS TO PATIENT SAFETY IN THE OFFICE

Medical errors can lead to patient harm in many ways in the outpatient setting. One of the earliest studies in this area looked at the incidence of adverse drug events in ambulatory practice.[7] Significant drug reactions were common, with almost one-third being found to be ameliorable or preventable. Another area of risk that has been identified is failure to review and follow up on outpatient test results.[8] Essentially any and all of the causes of preventable adverse events that can occur in the hospital can be found in the office setting, a fact confirmed by analysis of closed medical malpractice claims arising in ambulatory practice. Errors seen can include missed and delayed diagnosis,[9] wrong site/wrong procedure surgeries, and failure to recognize postoperative complications.[10]

Recently, several national organizations have publicly acknowledged the office as a clinical setting with significant risk for medical error and patient harm. In 2011 the American Medical Association released a 10-year review of ambulatory care, recognizing that:

> *Far more patients are cared for in ambulatory settings than are seen as inpatients; the harm that can occur in ambulatory settings is serious, and there are several ways in which the ambulatory setting is even more complex and prone to error than the inpatient setting.*[11]

The National Quality Forum has recently expanded its serious reportable events list to cover office-based settings.[12] Lastly, in 2013 the Agency for Healthcare Research and Quality issued a report on patient safety practices that strongly encouraged the use of several safety strategies with direct applicability to office practice, such as preoperative checklists, team training, and the use of simulation exercises in patient safety efforts.[13]

APPLICABILITY TO OFFICE PRACTICE IN OBSTETRICS AND GYNECOLOGY

Attention to office patient safety in obstetrics and gynecology actually predates the reports and reviews already outlined. Under the leadership of then president of the American College of Obstetricians and Gynecologists (ACOG), Dr Douglas Kirkpatrick, a task force was convened in 2008. Their charge was to develop recommendations to improve the safety of patient care in the obstetrics and gynecology (ob/gyn) office setting. The primary impetus to creating this task force was the steady migration of surgical procedures to the office that had once solely been performed in the hospital or ambulatory surgical center. This transition began with hysteroscopy in the 1980s and the loop electrocautery excision procedure in the 1990s, but has since progressed to include endometrial ablation for abnormal uterine bleeding and transcervical female sterilization procedures, in addition to many minor surgical procedures that had long been performed in ob/gyn offices such as suction curettage, vulvar cyst marsupialization, and various types of biopsies. These procedures sometimes involved analgesia/anesthesia ranging from injection of local anesthetic agents to administration of anxiolytic drugs and intravenous conscious sedation. As more complex procedures moved into the office setting, it was considered that safety standards that were routine in the operating room were not being brought into the office.

The work of this group was published in January 2010 as the Report of the Presidential Task Force on Patient Safety in the Office Setting.[14] It contained several general recommendations for improving safety in the ob/gyn office in general, but also more specifically in the performance of surgical procedures in the office. These concepts are expanded on in the following section and are briefly described here. The report advocated for the designation of an office medical director with responsibilities to ensure that all elements of patient safety were implemented and consistently executed. This action included maintaining appropriate credentialing and privileging of all physicians in the practice, including methodologies to determine ongoing competence in office surgical procedures. The medical director would also maintain an office policy and procedure manual that would include reference to such areas as informed consent and patients' rights. Specific to office surgery, the report called for the use of time-outs before office surgical procedures similar to what should be routinely done in hospital operating rooms, as well as the use of checklists. A sample checklist was provided (**Box 1**) that included elements to be addressed preoperatively, intraoperatively, postoperatively, and at the time of discharge from the office. The safe use of anesthesia was recognized as an area for concern, specifically the ability to rescue patients from excessive sedation. To this end, the periodic performance of mock drills was advocated, which would address not only rescue from overdoses of anesthetic medications but also vasovagal episodes, allergic reaction, cardiac events, respiratory arrest, and uterine hemorrhage. Lastly, it was recommended that a system be implemented to track surgical outcomes to allow for monitoring and continuous quality improvement. The principal objectives of the report were encapsulated in the so-called Seven Starter Steps to Office Patient Safety (**Box 2**).

While this task force on office safety was completing its work, a second workgroup was convened by ACOG to examine other elements of office safety in addition to those related to surgical procedures. This group was asked to develop an evaluation survey tool for assessing patient safety in office-based women's health care, and to collect data from ob/gyn physicians on gaps in knowledge and practice relative to these areas. The efforts of this group led to the development of ACOG's Office Patient Safety Assessment (OPSA) tool. This survey contained elements similar to those advocated in the Presidential Task Force Report regarding procedural safety, but in addition looked at 3 other important areas: safety culture in the office, practice management including record keeping, and medication safety. This survey was administered to 61 separate ob/gyn office sites, ranging in size from 1 to 26 providers with distribution across the United States. The results were published as a formal ACOG report in 2012.[15] The major areas of potential deficiencies in safety programs among these clinical ambulatory practices were identified. These areas included having a mechanism to grant surgical privileges in the office as well as ongoing monitoring of competency for procedures, performance of quarterly drills for response to untoward events, logging of all medication samples dispensed, and tracking of whether patients referred to other physicians were actually seen and a report received.

Armed with this information, ACOG decided that it would be feasible to transform OPSA into a more robust program of evaluating the safety climate and activities of ob/gyn offices across the country. This program would also feature the ability of individual offices to achieve a certification status in patient safety to be granted by ACOG's parallel organization, the American Congress of Obstetricians and Gynecologists. Even more importantly, public transparency for this program would be achieved by providing listing of certified offices through a dedicated Web site accessible to patients and other interested parties.[16] Thus was developed ACOG's Safety Certification for Outpatient Practice Excellence, known by the acronym of SCOPE. Similar to its

Box 1
Office surgical safety checklist

Office Surgical Safety Checklist

Patient Name: ____________ Primary Diagnosis: ____________ Date: ____________

Date of Birth: ____________ Procedure: ____________

Preoperative (Before Anesthesia/Analgesia)

- ______ ☐ Patient identity, site (marked), procedure, and consent confirmed
- ______ ☐ Current history and physical on chart
- ______ ☐ All medications taken previously that day reviewed and recorded
- ______ ☐ Patient's escort driver confirmed
- ______ ☐ No change in medical condition since last office visit, if changed, indicate here: ______
- ______ ☐ *Nil per os* (nothing by mouth—NPO) status confirmed
- ______ ☐ Preoperative instructions followed confirmed by patient
- ______ ☐ Known allergies reviewed
- ______ ☐ Any indicated lab work confirmed (eg, glucose level assessment in a diabetic patient or pregnancy test)
- ______ ☐ Preoperative vital signs documented
- ______ ☐ Pulse oximeter on the patient and functioning
- ______ ☐ Airway or aspiration risk assessed
- ______ ☐ Anesthesia and medication check is complete
- ______ ☐ Essential imaging is displayed

Preoperative (Before Incision)

- ______ ☐ Time-out (provider/patient/site/procedure)
- ______ ☐ Antibiotic prophylaxis given within 60 minutes of incision
- ______ ☐ Critical events anticipated:
  - ______ ☐ Critical or nonroutine steps
  - ______ ☐ Anticipated blood loss
  - ______ ☐ Sterility
  - ______ ☐ How long case will take
  - ______ ☐ Patient specific concerns
  - ______ ☐ Equipment issues

Intraoperative

- ______ ☐ Intraoperative medications recorded
- ______ ☐ If sedation implemented, oxygen saturation, blood pressure, pulse, and level of alertness monitored and documented every 5 minutes
- ______ ☐ For hysteroscopic procedures:
  - ______ ☐ Cavity assessment recorded per manufacturer's guidelines
  - ______ ☐ Fluid balance documented

Postoperative

- ______ ☐ Instrument, sponge, and needle counts completed
- ______ ☐ Specimen labeling confirmed
- ______ ☐ Equipment problems documented
- ______ ☐ Key concerns for recovery and management of patient documented

Discharge

- ______ ☐ Vital signs recorded and returned to within 20% of baseline
- ______ ☐ Adequate level of consciousness, pain control, ability to tolerate liquids by mouth, and ability to void (if appropriate for the procedure) documented
- ______ ☐ Discharge instruction sheet that includes how to recognize a postoperative emergency and steps to follow should one occur after discharge (eg, hemorrhage) discussed and given to patient
- ______ ☐ Appropriate postoperative follow-up appointment scheduled
- ______ ☐ Complications recorded
- ______ ☐ Follow-up call 24–48 hours after procedure assigned

predecessor OPSA, SCOPE requires office practices to submit information on office management and administration, documentation and reporting, medication safety, office-based surgical procedures, equipment, and quality improvement and measurement. In addition, there are currently modules related to nonmedically indicated delivery scheduling and smoking cessation. Additional modules are planned for the future.

Box 2
Seven starter steps to office patient safety

1. Designate a medical director with specific patient safety responsibilities
2. Create a specific short training manual for all office staff
    a. Import local hospital and ambulatory surgical center documents already available
    b. Contact state and other regulatory bodies for requirements that must be met in your locale
    c. Make this document available and mandatory reading with sign-offs by all staff
3. Create and perform a mock drill (try to do one every quarter, including one for cardiopulmonary resuscitation)
4. Create a checklist for one procedure and follow it closely; revise as needed
5. Survey and certify staff (who has basic life support or advanced cardiac life support training?)
6. Carefully reexamine anesthesia and analgesia methods and compare with published guidelines
7. Discuss patient safety goals with each patient to create a safer environment for the procedure

After review of submitted materials, an on-site validation survey is conducted by a specially trained physician reviewer. The purpose of this survey is simply to confirm the veracity of the previously submitted materials. An important feature of the SCOPE program is that it looks solely at processes of care in the office setting that contribute to the safe delivery of care. It does not look at outcomes of care or any other measures of the quality of the care provided. However, the SCOPE program is the current state of the art of assessment for office patient safety in ob/gyn. The remainder of this article looks in more depth at the areas addressed by this certification methodology.

COMPONENTS OF OFFICE SAFETY

Leadership

Like the Presidential Task Force report, the SCOPE survey tool begins with establishing the existence of a medical director responsible for patient safety issues. Leadership is a critical foundation on which an office safety program needs to be established. In a solo practitioner office, the physician is by default the medical director for patient safety. In a multi-physician office, however, taking the position that all physicians are responsible for patient safety is in fact equivalent to saying that no physicians in the office are responsible for patient safety. Most, if not all of the items that follow require that someone oversee the establishment of these safety processes and assure that they are consistently applied. A safety manual will need to be adopted, credentialing and privileging documents will need to be reviewed, and periodic staff meetings will need to be held to allow review of possible safety gaps, vulnerabilities, and near misses that have occurred. These aspects require dedicated time by a strong physician leader with a commitment to patient safety in the office. Consistent with this is the recognition by the practice as a whole that this time is valuable, and deserves either compensatory time off from other clinical duties or additional remuneration for the additional effort. Failure to do so will usually lead to haphazard oversight of important safety activities and a vulnerability of the practice's patients to adverse events.

Policy and Procedure Manual

One of the first responsibilities of the office medical director would be to establish a policy and procedure manual for the office, which is focused on safe clinical practices. This manual serves as a repository of various consent forms, checklists, preoperative and postoperative instructions, and other documents that are crucial to patient safety efforts. Absence of such a document was one of the safety gaps identified in the original OPSA surveys. Many office practices may find it difficult to establish such a manual where one has not existed. To this end, a model policy and procedure manual for ob/gyn practice is being developed for posting on the SCOPE Web site.[17] The table of contents alone would allow most practices to begin to develop their own set of documents (**Box 3**). Initial populating of the manual can be done from existing office documents or by adapting those in use at a local hospital or ambulatory surgical center where the physicians currently perform procedures. This document needs to be dynamic. There needs to be review and updating of all sections occurring on a regular schedule, with a 2-year cycle being a commonly chosen interval.

Credentialing and Privileging

When physicians join the medical staff of a hospital, they undergo a vetting process that includes both credentialing and privileging, and it is important to understand the distinction between these 2 concepts. Credentialing is making sure that people

Box 3
Model policy and procedure manual

- The purpose of a policy and procedure manual
- The role of the medical director
- Credentialing, privileging, scope of practice
- Quality improvement and peer review
- General policies and procedures for office-based surgery
- Scheduling procedure
- Preoperative notification and perioperative instructions
- Informed consent
- Anesthesia policies and procedures
- Perioperative checklists
- Safe culture policies and procedures
- Safety meetings, patient safety goals, reporting unsafe practices, creating a safe practice environment
- Medication management
- Medication review, logs, tracking, communication, teach-back techniques
- Patient communication, rights, privacy
- Patient rights and privacy policies, reporting rights violations, phone triage, email policies and procedures
- Tracking policies and procedures
- Laboratory findings, pathology, referrals
- Emergency management and drills

are indeed who they purport to be, through the verification of medical school graduation, residency completion, and the evaluation of state licensure records and letters of recommendation. It includes periodic reevaluation and notification of any material changes that ensue. Privileging, on the other hand, is the establishment of competency to perform specific procedures based on training and experience. Privileging may also include examination of the National Practitioner Data Bank to review malpractice history, and again should be subject to periodic reconfirmation. In a similar way, adherence to good patient safety practices requires that doctors in office practice undergo this type of process as well. This aspect is especially critical in practices where significant surgical procedures are performed. A sample office privileging document was appended to the Presidential Task Force Report (**Box 4**). Initial credentialing and privileging, periodic review, and record maintenance would be an important role of the office medical director. Similarly, nonclinical staff should have their training, licensing, and certifications verified at the time of hire and be periodically reconfirmed. Nonclinical staff should only perform those functions that fall within their scope of

Box 4
Sample privileging form

Sample Privileging Form

(sheet 1)

This sample application for privileges is provided for educational purposes only. It may require modification for use in a particular facility.

Outpatient Privileging

Delineation for Privileges for: ________ **Credentialing Period:** ________

Practice Name: ________ **Department:** ________ **Specialty:** ________

Clinical Category	Procedure Description	Approximate Volume in Prior Year	Amount Required	Requested	Inpatient Privileges Y N N/A	Medical Director Approval Y N N/A
Cervix						
	LEEP	______	______	☐		
	Colposcopy cervix	______	______	☐		
	Laser therapy[a]	______	______	☐		
	Other:	______	______	☐		
Contraception						
	IUD insertion	______	______	☐		
	IUD removal	______	______	☐		
	Tubal ligation[a]	______	______	☐		
	Other:	______	______	☐		
Diagnostic Gyn ultrasound	Gyn U/S	______	______	☐		
	Sonohysteroscopy	______	______	☐		
	Other:	______	______	☐		
Diagnostic Ob ultrasound	3rd trimester OB U/S	______	______	☐		
	1st trimester OB U/S	______	______	☐		
	Other:	______	______	☐		
Excision of lesion						
	Excision of lesion trunk or exrm	______	______	☐		
	Excision of lesion genitalia	______	______	☐		
	Other:	______	______	☐		

Abbreviations: exrm, extremity; IUD, intrauterine device; LEEP, loop electrosurgical excision procedure; U/S, ultrasound.

[a] Denotes that procedure requires documentation of performance competency in an inpatient surgical setting prior to performing in an outpatient office setting.

Sample Privileging Form

(sheet 2)

Outpatient Privileging

Delineation for Privileges for:________________ **Credentialing Period:**________________

Practice Name:________________ **Department:**________________ **Specialty:**________________

Clinical Category	Procedure Description	Approximate Volume in Prior Year	Amount Required	Requested	Inpatient Privileges Y N N/A	Medical Director Approval Y N N/A
Needle aspiration						
	Needle aspiration of breast cyst	______	______	☐		
NST						
	Nonstress test	______	______	☐		
Pessary						
	Pessary fitting	______	______	☐		
Uterus						
	Endometrial biopsy	______	______	☐		
	D&C[a]	______	______	☐		
	Hysterosalpingogram	______	______	☐		
	Hysteroscopy[a]	______	______	☐		
	Ablation[a]	______	______	☐		
	Other:	______	______	☐		
Vagina						
	Destruction of vaginal lesion	______	______	☐		
	Vaginal biopsy	______	______	☐		
	Laser therapy[a]	______	______	☐		
	Colposcopy vagina[a]	______	______	☐		
	Other:	______	______	☐		
Vulvar						
	Destruction of vulva lesion	______	______	☐		
	Vulvar biopsy	______	______	☐		
	Laser therapy[a]	______	______	☐		
	Hymenotomy	______	______	☐		
	Perineoplasty	______	______	☐		
	I&D of vulva or perineal abscess	______	______	☐		
	Other:	______	______	☐		

Abbreviations: D&C, dilation and curettage; I&D, incision and drainage; NST, nonstress test.

[a]Denotes that procedure requires documentation of performance competency in an inpatient surgical setting prior to performing in an outpatient office setting.

practice as defined by such licensure and certification according to applicable state law.

Safety Culture

Although an in-depth discussion of the "culture of safety" or "just culture"[18] in health care organizations is beyond the scope of this article, the existence of such a culture in the office setting is another crucial element in reducing the risk of adverse events. At its heart, in this context a culture of safety is the recognition by everyone working in the office environment that patient safety is their primary responsibility. Part of this is the recognition of a duty to report unsafe practices, near misses, and actual adverse events as a learning tool to enable the office to enforce adherence to patient safety policies and, if necessary, revise or add to such policies to reduce opportunities for patient harm. The SCOPE survey recognizes the importance of a safety culture in several ways, all of which should be considered for adoption to maximize patient safety. All staff should be trained on a regular basis on patient safety issues relevant to the types of patients seen and procedures performed. Two patient identifiers, such as name and date of birth, should be used when any patient first registers at the reception desk for an office visit, and there should be a clear system in place to allow office staff to reach a physician if none is present in the office both during and outside regular office hours. There should be a mechanism for any physician or other staff member to report safety concerns to the medical director. Regular meetings should be held for all staff to have a forum to discuss any safety concerns, including breaches of safety policies observed, near misses, and actual adverse events. These meetings need to be conducted in a blame-free atmosphere that encourages this discussion without fear of retaliation, with the goal being adherence to policies and process improvement. Office personnel should be trained in basic life support, and be well versed in the office management plan for acute emergencies that may require summoning of emergency personnel, such as cardiac events or respiratory arrest. A useful adjunct to having a safety culture is to regularly assess it and monitor improvement as additional components are put in place through the use of a validated staff survey tool[19] that can be administered to clinical and nonclinical staff alike.

Documentation

Several elements of office documentation are important to patient safety, whether an electronic health record is utilized or not.[20] Most critical to patient safety is an adequate system that tracks laboratory, imaging, and cytology/pathology results to ensure that ordered tests are in fact performed, the results received, and the information conveyed to patients regarding both normal and abnormal results.[21] As discussed earlier, failure to track laboratory data is a significant source of missed or delayed diagnosis, patient harm, and subsequent malpractice litigation. In a similar way, it is necessary to have a system in place to track referrals from the office to outside specialists, such as a referral to a general surgeon after an abnormal mammogram. This system needs to include the ability to track whether the consultation in fact took place, and if a report from the consultant was received back in the office and communicated to the patient. Such tracking applies equally to patients referred to the office from outside physicians, to confirm that the referral was acknowledged, a report was submitted to the referring physician, and that the patient understands the proposed plan of care. There needs to be a system in place to remind patients of upcoming appointments and to review all "no-show" patient records, to ensure that important screening tests or follow-up management decisions are not missed. All communications from patients, such as telephone calls and, potentially, emails, should be incorporated into the medical record to include date, time, and information provided. If communication with patients occurs by email or other electronic means, it is crucial that this only be done through secure portals that protect patient privacy.

Medication Safety

This area of patient safety is not specifically addressed in the Presidential Task Force Report, but has been clearly recognized as a source of patient harm in the office setting. All medications, including over-the-counter drugs, vitamins, and herbal preparations, and all allergies should be listed in the medical record. The medication and allergy list should be specifically reviewed and updated at every office visit. This record keeping is probably an office's best defense against adverse drug reactions, especially in the increasingly common electronic health record environment.

Complete and correct recording of drugs and allergies are required to trigger appropriate alerts warning of inappropriate drug prescription or drug incompatibilities. A special consideration in the ob/gyn office setting is caution regarding prescription of contraindicated drugs to pregnant patients, and these considerations should be incorporated into any automatic alert system. Use of so-called e-prescribing or auto-fax systems will decrease the possibility of misreading of handwritten prescriptions and wrong dispensing of sound-alike drugs at the pharmacy. Another aspect of medication safety is appropriate storage and dispensing of injectable medications, sample drugs, and emergency drugs. All drugs stored in the office should be appropriately secured, and periodically checked for expiration dates to allow discarding and replacement as required. When injectable medications or sample drugs are dispensed, a log should be kept to record patient name, medication name, date dispensed, expiration date, and lot number. The latter allows notification of patients if a manufacturer's recall is ever issued that affects a sample medication the office has stocked. An increasingly recognized aspect of medication safety in the office involves how patients are instructed in the use of newly prescribed medications.[22] Communication with patients in general should always try to take into account their level of health literacy[23] in terms of their ability to understand what is being imparted to them, whether it is in the form of verbal or written instructions. When discussing medications, a valuable technique that takes health literacy into account is the teach-back method, when a physician instructs a patient in the appropriate use of a medication, then asks the patient to in turn "teach" the physician how to take the medication correctly. Use of this technique can improve patient compliance and correct medication usage.[24] Lastly, similarly to teach-back, whenever a medication order is transmitted orally to a staff member by a physician, the staff member should repeat the order out loud back to the physician, thus ensuring that the information has been correctly conveyed to the staff member and in turn to the patient.

Surgical Procedures

It is important when performing surgery in the office setting that only those patients be operated on whose general medical condition makes it safe for them to undergo a procedure. The most appropriate method to evaluate this is through the American Society of Anesthesiologists Physical Status classification system.[25] For the most part, office surgical procedures should be limited to those patients in category I or II, meaning those that are either completely healthy or those with mild systemic disease that does not limit physical activity. Unless an anesthesiologist or nurse anesthetist is used to monitor the patient under deep sedation, patients undergoing office surgery should be limited to minimal or moderate sedation. Minimal sedation, or anxiolysis, is a drug-induced state characterized by the ability to respond normally to verbal commands. Safely providing even this level of anesthesia requires the presence of someone trained in basic life support to be present with the patient until discharge, and ready availability of equipment for cardiorespiratory support and treatment of anaphylaxis. Moderate sedation, or conscious sedation, is a drug-induced state whereby consciousness is depressed, but the patient spontaneously maintains adequate ventilation and responds purposefully to verbal commands or light tactile stimulation. Safe administration of this level of anesthesia in the office requires the presence of a licensed physician and another health professional trained in advanced cardiac life support until the patient is discharged. Equipment for cardiorespiratory support and treatment of anaphylaxis should be immediately available. Patients should always be required to have a friend or adult family member available to escort them home after any office procedure during which any form of sedation is used. Patients should be contacted by phone or secure email 48 hours after any office surgical procedure to make sure that they have not suffered any complications or other ill effects, and to answer any questions they may have.

Patients should be given written preoperative and postoperative instructions, which should adhere to principles of health literacy discussed earlier. Instructions should be written at a reading level that is comprehensible to the majority of patients, and should make minimal use of technical terms or medical jargon. Instructions should be available in multiple languages as appropriate for the patient population being served. Similarly, informed consent should be documented before any surgical procedure, to include a discussion of risks, benefits, complications, and alternatives.[26] Informed consent is not simply having a patient read and sign a preprinted form, but must include discussion of the aforementioned issues, with the patient being given an opportunity to ask questions. The patient's medical record should contain confirmation that this discussion took place.

As already discussed, a checklist should be used for all office procedures; a sample from the Presidential Task Force Report is shown in **Box 1**. The use of checklists has become recognized as a critical element in reducing patient harm during surgical procedures. Ideal checklists should fit on one side of a printed page, should be limited to as few items as possible for each relevant activity, and should consist only of those crucial elements that could lead to failure and harm if omitted.[27] The sample checklist provided meets all such elements, with the activities related to the performance of office surgery broken down into the areas of preanesthesia, before initiation of procedure, intraoperatively, postoperatively, and at the time of discharge. One of the items is a surgical time-out, which is a pause before starting the procedure to make sure that the correct patient is present and the correct procedure planned. It is an important that this safety practice be performed before even minor office procedures, as well as confirming the absence of pregnancy before any procedure with the potential to harm or interrupt an early gestation.

True medical emergencies in the office or related to office surgeries are rare, but patient safety demands that the physicians and other staff be fully prepared to handle these emergencies if they arise. The procedure on how to deal with emergencies should be incorporated into the office policy manual and reviewed with staff on a regular basis. The best way to prepare is to hold mock drills, with one drill per quarter being a reasonable interval. These drills should be rotated to include the most uncommon but serious problems that might be encountered, including respiratory arrest, myocardial infarction, major hemorrhage, syncope/vasovagal reaction, and fire. The Presidential Task Force Report includes recommendations on how to manage most of these issues and how to conduct drills to prepare for their possible occurrence.

Equipment Safety

The maintenance, cleaning, and sterilization of office surgical equipment is the last element addressed in the SCOPE process, and one that is clearly important in preventing injury and infection in patients. Office staff should be trained in the correct use of surgical equipment, and should always follow the manufacturer's recommendations for periodic testing for its function and safety. For reusable equipment, proper cleansing and sterilization policies should be established and followed, again according to manufacturer's recommendations if appropriate. For any emergency medications or cardiorespiratory support equipment in the office, physicians and staff should know their location, train in their use using mock drills, and be sure that expiration dates are regularly checked.

Other Considerations

Not addressed in the SCOPE application is the issue of physician fatigue. This aspect may have particular applicability to ob/gyn office practice, in that many physicians have had the experience of being up all night on call and then going on to a full day of office practice, possibly including the performance of office surgical procedures. It is now recognized that sleep deprivation can significantly affect judgment and reaction times.[28,29] Being awake for 19 to 21 consecutive hours yields cognitive performance scores equal to those observed with blood ethanol levels consistent with legal intoxication.[30] With the movement of greater numbers of more complex surgical procedures into the office setting, physicians should consider the wisdom of scheduling such procedures at times when there may be a risk of a fatigued operator.

SUMMARY

While it is laudable that much effort is being directed toward patient safety in hospitals, far more care is provided on an annual basis in physicians' offices.[31] There are clear vulnerabilities to adverse events and patient harm in this setting, even more so for ob/gyn physicians who are performing increasingly complex surgical procedures in this setting. Fortunately, ACOG and other safety-minded organizations are now recognizing these vulnerabilities and are providing road maps for safer care. Physicians in this specialty should embrace all the elements of office practice and surgical care outlined in this article, with the clear goal being to reduce the chances of their patients suffering the consequences of adverse events.

REFERENCES

1. National Research Council. To err is human: building a safer health system. Washington, DC: The National Academies Press; 2000.
2. National Research Council. Crossing the quality chasm: a new health system for the 21st century. Washington, DC: The National Academies Press; 2001.
3. Leape LL, Berwick DM. Five years after to err is human: what have we learned? JAMA 2005;293(19):2384–90.
4. Reason JT. Managing the risk of organizational accidents. Farnham (United Kingdom): Ashgate Publishing Co; 1997.
5. Veltman LL. Getting to Havarti: moving toward patient safety in obstetrics. Obstet Gynecol 2007;110(5):1146–50.
6. Baron RJ. Patient safety: a perspective from office practice. AHRQ Web M&M. 2009. Available at: http://webmm.ahrq.gov/perspective.aspx?perspectiveID=75. Accessed May 24, 2013.
7. Gandhi TK, Weingart SN, Borus J, et al. Adverse drug events in ambulatory care. N Engl J Med 2003;348(16):1556–64.
8. Poon EG, Gandhi TK, Sequist TD, et al. "I wish I had seen this test result earlier!": dissatisfaction with test result management systems in primary care. Arch Intern Med 2004;164:2223–8.
9. Gandhi TK, Kachalia A, Thomas EJ, et al. Missed and delayed diagnoses in the ambulatory setting: a study of closed malpractice claims. Ann Intern Med 2006; 145(7):488–96.
10. Rapp C. Reducing malpractice risk by preventing medical errors. Presentation at Medical Group Management Association meeting. Chicago, April 22, 2013.

11. Lorincz CY, Drazen E, Sokol PE, et al. Research in ambulatory patient safety 2000-2010: a ten-year review. Chicago (IL): American Medical Association; 2011. Available at: www.ama-assn.org/go/patient safety.
12. National Quality Forum (NQF). Serious reportable events in healthcare—2011 update: a consensus report. Washington, DC: NQF; 2011.
13. Shekelle PG, Wachter RM, Pronovost PJ, et al. Making patients safer II: an update critical analysis of the evidence for patient safety practices. Review no 211 AHRQ Publication No. 13-E001-EF. Rockville (MD): Agency for Healthcare Research and Quality; 2013.
14. Erickson TB, Kirkpatrick DH, DeFrancesco MS, et al. Executive summary of the American College of Obstetricians and Gynecologists Presidential Task Force on Patient Safety in the Office Setting: reinvigorating safety in office-based gynecologic surgery. Obstet Gynecol 2010;115(1):147–51.
15. American College of Obstetricians and Gynecologists. Office patient safety assessment: national results report. 2012. Available at: http://www.scopeforwomenshealth.org/ckfinder/userfiles/files/OPSA%20Results%20National%20Report%20-%20April%202012.pdf. Accessed May 24, 2013.
16. American College of Obstetricians and Gynecologists. SCOPE home page. Available at: www.scopeforwomenshealth.org. Accessed May 24, 2013.
17. American College of Obstetricians and Gynecologists. SCOPE Policies and Procedures Guide. Available at: http://www.scopeforwomenshealth.org/ckfinder/userfiles/files/PPManualMJS.pdf. Accessed May 24, 2013.
18. Marx D. Patient safety and the "just culture": a primer for health care executives. New York: Columbia University; 2001.
19. Pronovost P, Sexton B. Assessing safety culture: guidelines and recommendations. Qual Saf Health Care 2005;14:231–3.
20. American College of Obstetricians and Gynecologists. Patient safety and the electronic health record. Committee opinion no. 472. Obstet Gynecol 2010;116:1245–7.
21. American College of Obstetricians and Gynecologists. Tracking and reminder systems. Committee opinion no. 546. Obstet Gynecol 2012;120:1535–7.
22. American College of Obstetricians and Gynecologists. Partnering with patients to improve safety. Committee opinion no. 490. Obstet Gynecol 2011;117:1247–9.
23. American College of Obstetricians and Gynecologists. Health literacy. Committee opinion no. 491. Obstet Gynecol 2011;117:1250–3.
24. American College of Obstetricians and Gynecologists. Effective patient-physician communication. Committee opinion no. 492. Obstet Gynecol 2011;117:1254–7.
25. American Society of Anesthesiologist. Physical status classification system. Available at: http://www.asahq.org/Home/For-Members/Clinical-Information/ASA-Physical-Status-Classification-System. Accessed May 26, 2013.
26. American College of Obstetricians and Gynecologists. Informed consent. Committee opinion no. 439. Obstet Gynecol 2009;114:401–8.
27. Gawande A. The checklist manifesto: how to get things right. London: Picador; 2011.
28. American College of Obstetricians and Gynecologists. Patient safety in the surgical environment. Committee opinion no. 464. Obstet Gynecol 2010;116:786–90.
29. American College of Obstetricians and Gynecologists. Fatigue and patient safety. Committee opinion no. 519. Obstet Gynecol 2012;119:683–5.
30. Clark S. Sleep deprivation: implications for obstetric practice in the United States. Am J Obstet Gynecol 2009;201:136.e1–4.
31. Stumpf PG. Practical solutions to improve patient safety in the obstetrics/gynecology office setting and in the operating room. Obstet Gynecol Clin North Am 2008; 35:18–35.

Pain Relief for Obstetric and Gynecologic Ambulatory Procedures

Rebecca H. Allen, MD, MPH[a,*], Elizabeth Micks, MD, MPH[b], Alison Edelman, MD, MPH[c]

KEYWORDS

• Pain • Paracervical block • IUD • Hysteroscopy • Endometrial biopsy • Colposcopy • Uterine aspiration • Ambulatory

KEY POINTS

- Pain control in the ambulatory setting should be multimodal and include both pharmacologic and nonpharmacologic interventions.
- The provision of even minimal sedation (anxiolysis) and local anesthesia in the office requires emergency medication availability and protocols.
- Misoprostol does not reduce pain for office gynecologic procedures.
- Paracervical block is effective in reducing the pain of cervical dilation and uterine aspiration.

INTRODUCTION

Increasingly, minor gynecologic procedures are moving from operating rooms to the office. In this setting, providers often perform these procedures without the assistance of a nurse anesthetist or anesthesiologist. Therefore, it is important for clinicians to be aware of the safety and efficacy of different pain control regimens. The goal of most office-based procedures is twofold: (1) to be able to safely and successfully perform the procedure, and (2) patient comfort. Obviously, patient comfort directly affects the ability to safely complete a procedure, and not all women are candidates for an office procedure with limited options for pain control. Providers should screen each patient to ensure she is appropriate for and can tolerate an office-based procedure. In addition, certain conditions preclude an ambulatory procedure, such as an anxiety disorder, a high-risk airway, obesity, or other medical problems. This article outlines

[a] Department of Obstetrics and Gynecology, Warren Alpert Medical School of Brown University, Women & Infants Hospital, 101 Dudley Street, Providence, RI 02905, USA; [b] Department of Obstetrics and Gynecology, University of Washington, Box 356460, Seattle, WA 98195-6460, USA; [c] Department of Obstetrics and Gynecology, Oregon Health & Science University, 3181 Southwest Sam Jackson, UHN 50, Portland, OR 97239, USA
* Corresponding author.
E-mail address: rhallen@wihri.org

Obstet Gynecol Clin N Am 40 (2013) 625–645
http://dx.doi.org/10.1016/j.ogc.2013.08.005
0889-8545/13/$ – see front matter

effective pain control regimens based on the published evidence for the most common gynecologic procedures performed in the office.

ANATOMY OF PAIN

The internal female reproductive organs are innervated by 2 main pathways (**Fig. 1**). The fundus of the uterus is innervated by sympathetic fibers from T10 to L2 via the inferior hypogastric plexus, which enters the uterus by the uterosacral ligaments, and by nerves from the ovarian plexuses at the cornua.[1] The upper vagina, cervix, and lower uterine segment are innervated by parasympathetic fibers from S2 to S4, which enter the cervix along with the uterine blood vessels at 3 o'clock and 9 o'clock. The lower vagina and vulva are supplied by the pudendal nerve (S2, S3, and S4).

CHARACTERISTICS ASSOCIATED WITH PAIN

The experience of pain is influenced not only by physical factors but also by psychological and social factors. Regardless of procedure type, anxiety, depression, and a woman's anticipation of the pain she will experience are strong predictors of the pain experienced during office gynecologic procedures.[2–5] For procedures that involve cervical dilation and the passage of a device or cannula through the internal os of the cervix, a history of dysmenorrhea, nulliparity, and postmenopausal status are associated with increased pain.[1,6,7] Previous vaginal birth, more so than cesarean delivery, is associated with decreased pain.[4]

SAFE USE OF ANALGESIA AND ANESTHESIA

Safe use of anesthesia in the office setting requires careful planning as individuals vary in their response to these medications and the level of sedation can change rapidly (**Table 1**). Providers must be able to manage patients who experience deeper than intended levels of sedation.[8] Thus, the use of anesthesia in the office requires an understanding of state and hospital-specific regulations, advanced life-support training, availability of monitoring and resuscitation equipment, and an emergency referral system. Although less stringent requirements may be required when providing oral versus intravenous sedative medications, both routes can cause similar levels of sedation and risks.

Although the level of sedation is often a continuum, it has been defined into the categories of minimal, moderate, and deep sedation (see **Table 1**). Office-based anesthesia is typically limited to the provision of moderate sedation or less, but most providers restrict their practice to minimal sedation using a combination of oral anxiolytics and analgesics with local anesthesia. Minimal sedation or anxiolysis is defined as a drug-induced state during which patients respond normally to verbal commands. Although cognitive function and coordination may be impaired, ventilation and cardiovascular functions are not affected. Personnel with training in Basic Life Support and emergency equipment for cardiorespiratory support and treatment of anaphylaxis should be available even at this level of sedation.

Moderate sedation (formerly conscious sedation) is defined as a drug-induced depression of consciousness during which patients respond purposefully to verbal commands, either alone or accompanied by light tactile stimulation. Providing moderate sedation in the office requires higher levels of equipment and monitoring as well as requirements for personnel skill levels and training (Advanced Cardiac Life Support).

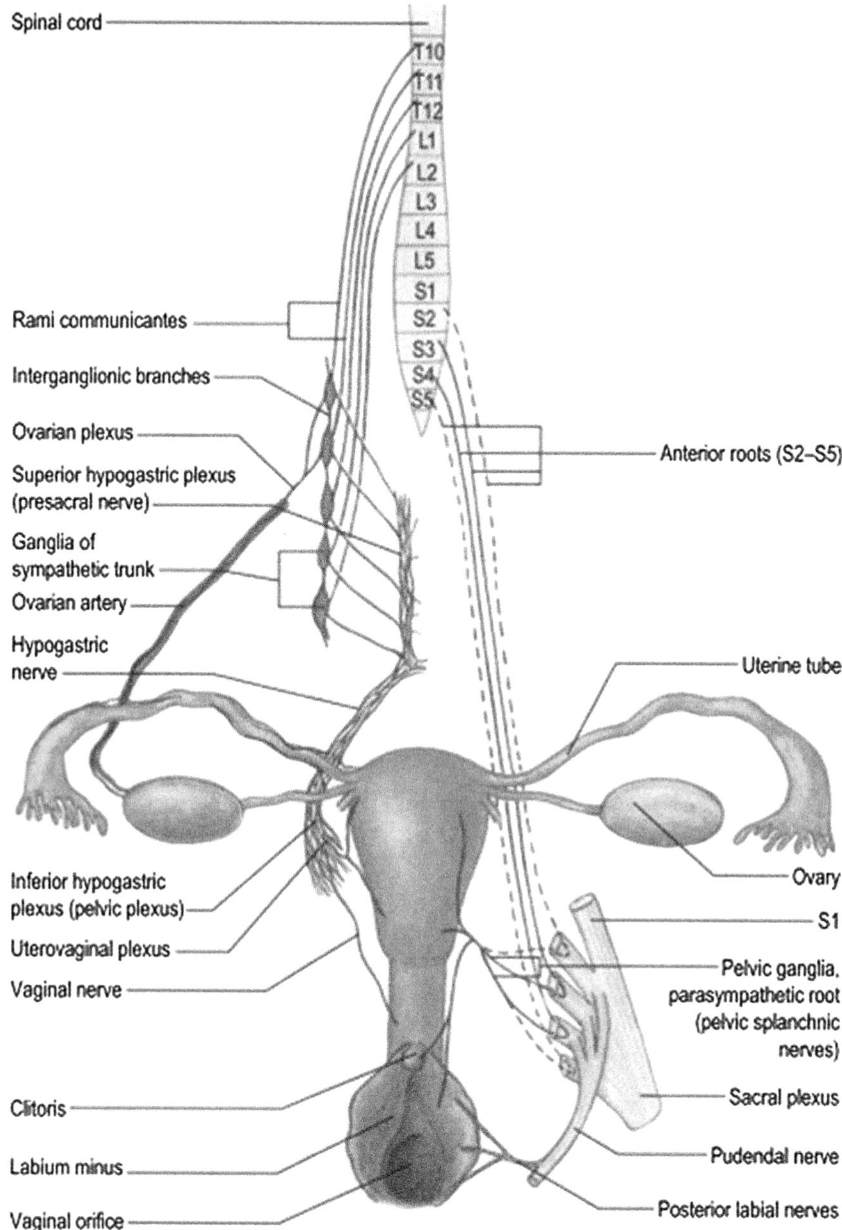

Fig. 1. Innervation of the female reproductive system. (*From* Standring S. Gray's anatomy: the anatomical basis of clinical practice. 40th edition. Edinburgh (United Kingdom): Churchill Livingstone/Elsevier; 2008; with permission.)

Analgesia

Nonsteroidal antiinflammatory drugs (NSAIDs) such as ibuprofen decrease uterine activity and pain by inhibiting cyclooxygenase and thereby reducing circulating prostaglandins. These drugs have been effective in decreasing pain in some gynecologic

Table 1
Definition of general anesthesia and levels of sedation/analgesia

	Minimal Sedation/ Anxiolysis	Moderate Conscious Sedation	Deep Sedation	General Anesthesia
Responsiveness	Normal response to verbal stimulation	Purposeful response to verbal or tactile stimulation	Purposeful response after repeated or painful stimulation	Unarousable even with painful stimulus
Airway	Unaffected	No intervention required	Intervention may be required	Intervention often required
Spontaneous ventilation	Unaffected	Adequate	May be inadequate	Frequently inadequate
Cardiovascular function	Unaffected	Usually maintained	Usually maintained	May be impaired

Data from Continuum of depths of sedation: definition of general anesthesia and levels of sedation/analgesia. American Society of Anesthesiologists. Available at: http://www.asahq.org. Accessed September 5, 2013.

procedures, especially, postoperatively. Common NSAIDs used include ibuprofen, naproxen, diclofenac, and ketorolac. Like NSAIDs, acetaminophen also inhibits the enzyme cyclooxygenase, however its action is in the central nervous system rather than the periphery. This medication is often combined with opioids, but may also be used alone. It is metabolized hepatically and may be safely used along with NSAIDs, although there is no evidence this combination is more effective. Acetaminophen is inferior to ibuprofen for uterine pain, however, it is an option for women who cannot tolerate NSAIDs.[9]

Oral opioids are widely available in different forms (ie, oxycodone, hydrocodone, codeine). Analgesia is produced primarily through interaction with endogenous opioid mu receptors. Fentanyl is a short-acting opioid that is 100 times more potent than morphine. Opioids provide analgesia and cause euphoria. Intravenous fentanyl is the most common opioid used for moderate sedation because of its rapid onset, brief duration, and lack of histamine release. Naloxone reverses fentanyl when dosed at 0.2 to 0.4 mg increments.

Anxiolysis

Benzodiazepines have anxiolytic, amnestic, anticonvulsant, and sedative properties. A common misperception is that they have a direct analgesic effect but they do not. For perioperative use, lorazepam, an intermediate-acting benzodiazepine, is generally preferable to the long-acting diazepam. Short-acting benzodiazepines such as midazolam have a half-life between 1 and 12 hours. Those that are intermediate acting have a half-life of 12 to 40 hours, and the long-acting benzodiazepines have half-lives of 40 to 250 hours. The long-acting medications have risks of accumulation, especially in elderly patients or those with hepatic impairment, but they have less risk of withdrawal and/or rebound effects. Many providers use 1 to 2 mg of lorazepam for anxiolysis.[1] Intravenous midazolam is often used as part of a moderate sedation regimen. Midazolam can be reversed with flumazenil dosed at 0.2 mg increments.

Combination Regimens

Benzodiazepines are often coadministered with opioids for intravenous (IV) sedation. When used concurrently, it is important to be aware of the risk of respiratory depression. The most common medications used for IV moderate sedation are midazolam (1–2 mg) and fentanyl (50–100 μg). When used together at these doses, midazolam and fentanyl provide excellent sedation with a good safety profile. One retrospective study of more than 1400 consecutive women who underwent first-trimester surgical abortions with a maximum dose of 2 mg of midazolam and 100 μg of fentanyl found that there were few complications reported (0.3%), none having to do with respiratory depression, and no hospital transfers.[10]

Local Anesthesia

Safe use of local anesthetics requires avoiding toxicity and understanding how to quickly recognize and manage complications. The most common local anesthetics used in the office are of the amide class, such as lidocaine or bupivacaine. Amides are associated with fewer allergic reactions and lower cost compared with the ester class (procaine and 2-chloroprocaine). The maximum dose of lidocaine without epinephrine should not exceed 4.5 mg/kg (**Table 2**).[11] A dose of 200 mg of lidocaine (20 mL of 1% lidocaine) is often used for paracervical block and is well below the threshold of toxicity.[1] At low serum levels of lidocaine, patients may experience tinnitus and numbness of the mouth. This is not uncommon when using paracervical blocks during pregnancy because of the vascularity of the cervix. At higher levels of lidocaine, patients may experience visual disturbances, confusion, seizure, or cardiorespiratory arrest. Techniques to lower the risk of lidocaine toxicity include adding vasopressin or epinephrine to reduce systemic absorption and aspirating before injecting to reduce the risk of intravascular instillation.[1] Although the paracervical block has been shown to be effective for many gynecologic procedures, the block itself causes considerable discomfort.[12] To lower the pain of lidocaine injections, many providers add sodium bicarbonate to buffer the acidity of the lidocaine (1 mL of 8.4% sodium bicarbonate to every 10 mL of anesthetic solution).[11] Other providers use dental syringes with anesthesia cartridges and 27-gauge needles to reduce the pain of injection. The administration of local anesthesia in gynecologic procedures can take different forms: topical, intracervical, paracervical, and intrauterine (**Fig. 2**).

Nonpharmacologic Techniques

It is important to offer nonpharmacologic methods of pain management in conjunction with medication regimens. Women manage pain best if they have been thoroughly

Table 2
Maximum allowable dose of local anesthetics for adults

Agent	Concentration (%)	Maximum Safe Dose (mg)	Maximum Volume (mL)
Lidocaine	0.5	300	60
	1	300	30
Bupivacaine	0.25	175	70
Lidocaine-epinephrine	0.5	500	100
	1	500	50
Bupivacaine-epinephrine	0.25	225	90

Data from Roberts J, Hedges J. Clinical procedures in emergency medicine. 5th edition. Chapter 29. Local and topical anesthesia. Philadelphia: Saunders; 2010.

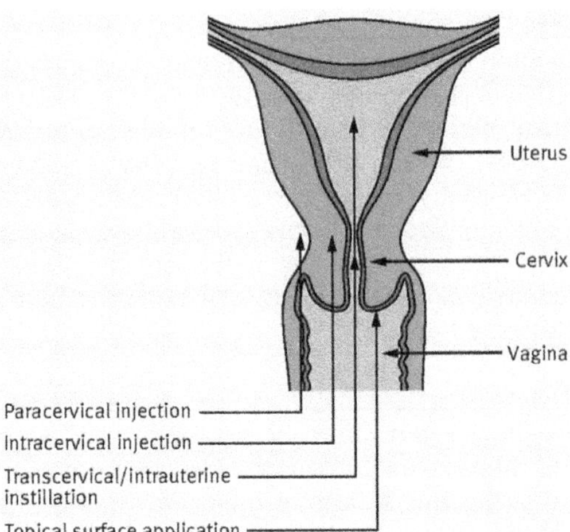

Fig. 2. Different methods of administration of local anesthetics. (*From* Cooper NA, Khan KS, Clark TJ. Local anesthesia for pain control during outpatient hysteroscopy: systematic review and meta-analysis. BMJ 2010;340:c1130; with permission.)

counseled and know what to expect in terms of procedural steps and time. Other techniques include music, positive suggestion, relaxation, and guided imagery.[13] Verbocaine or talking to the patient and distracting her throughout the procedure is also helpful.[1] Having a support person sit with the patient through the procedure can also be helpful. A heating pad can be helpful for uterine cramping.[14]

PAIN RELIEF FOR AMBULATORY PROCEDURES

Tenaculum Placement

In most gynecologic procedures involving cervical and uterine instrumentation, the single-toothed tenaculum is used for stabilization and traction, and allows descent of the uterus within the speculum. Most importantly, the tenaculum decreases the flexion of the uterus and eases passage of instruments into the endometrial cavity. Tenaculum placement generally precedes insertion of an intrauterine device (IUD), removal of lost IUDs, endometrial biopsy, uterine aspiration, and hysteroscopy. Few studies exist directly comparing methods to decrease pain with tenaculum placement; commonly described strategies include slow placement of the tenaculum, having the patient cough while the tenaculum is placed, and/or application of local anesthetics. Some providers also choose to use atraumatic tenaculums although there are no data that these are less painful than the single-toothed tenaculum.

Topical local anesthetics seem to be somewhat effective for decreasing pain with single-tooth tenaculum placement depending on the medication, although studies are inconsistent with regard to the intervening wait time. A placebo-controlled randomized trial by Liberty and colleagues[15] demonstrated decreased pain with cervical instrumentation (tenaculum placement and cannula placement) with lidocaine-prilocaine cream applied via cervical cup 30 minutes before a hysterosalpingogram. However, this approach may be impractical in a busy office setting. In another placebo-controlled trial evaluating pain with tenaculum placement and other gynecologic procedures, Rabin and colleagues[16] showed decreased pain with 20% benzocaine gel applied 1 to 2 minutes before tenaculum placement. Approximately, 9% of patients in the active benzocaine group experienced pain versus 65% in the placebo group (P<.05). Benzocaine is an ester and therefore can be more allergenic than other topical agents. In contrast, a study evaluating 2% lidocaine gel for IUD insertion found no difference in pain with tenaculum placement after applying 0.5 to 1 mL of gel to the tenaculum site 3 minutes before the procedure.[17]

Topical anesthetic spray is another common approach. In a placebo-controlled trial of lidocaine spray before office hysteroscopy, Davies and colleagues[18] found that patients who received 10% lidocaine spray (3 metered sprays to the ectocervix 1 minute before) experienced significantly less pain with tenaculum placement compared with placebo (9.0 vs 18.5 mm on the visual analog scale). A comparative study by Zullo and colleagues[19] found that lidocaine-prilocaine cream was more effective than lidocaine spray for tenaculum placement, although in this case the cream was placed 10 minutes before the procedure, whereas the spray was applied immediately before. However, another study by Costello and colleagues[20] found no difference in pain scores with tenaculum placement when comparing spray or gel containing equivalent doses of lidocaine.

One of the more common techniques for minimizing pain with tenaculum placement is superficial injection of a small amount of local anesthetic into the anterior lip of the cervix. This is a convenient approach when a full paracervical block is also planned, and is described in several recent studies of pain with gynecologic procedures.[12,21] There are no placebo-controlled trials evaluating the efficacy of this technique, although there is some evidence that anesthetic injection does decrease pain with tenaculum placement. Robinson and colleagues[22] concluded that injection of 6 mL of lidocaine circumferentially around the cervix before hysterosalpingogram was more effective than saline injection or no injection for decreasing pain with the tenaculum. In addition, 2 mL of 1% lidocaine decreased pain during tenaculum placement in a trial evaluating paracervical block for IUD insertion.[23]

Most effective method of pain relief for tenaculum placement

- Intracervical injection of local anesthetic

Colposcopy and Cervical Biopsies

Many women find colposcopy with the application of dilute acetic acid, cervical biopsies, and endocervical curettage (ECC) uncomfortable. Providers vary on whether they choose to anesthetize the cervix and upper vagina for biopsies. However, local anesthesia is essential for biopsies of the lower vagina and vulva. As with other gynecologic procedures, baseline anxiety, nulliparity, and history of dysmenorrhea are predictors of pain during colposcopy.

A double-blind, placebo-controlled, randomized controlled trial (RCT) evaluated 800 mg of ibuprofen 30 minutes before colposcopy, 2 mL of 20% benzocaine topical gel, both treatments, or neither treatment.[24] Women (n = 99) were randomized to 1 of the 4 arms. There were no differences between the 4 groups in terms of mean pain with cervical biopsy or ECC. The median overall pain score with cervical biopsy and ECC was 2.75 out of 10 and 3.5 out of 10, respectively. Other topical anesthetics have likewise been ineffective in reducing pain with cervical biopsy and ECC.[25,26]

Similar to tenaculum placement, the infiltration of local anesthetic before cervical biopsy during colposcopy has been investigated. Although the trial was not blinded, 0.5 mL of 1% lidocaine with a 27- gauge needle decreased pain compared with no injection in 1 study of 56 women (mean pain score 0–10, 1.2 vs 4.0, P<.001).[27] There are concerns, however, that anesthetic injection prolongs the procedure, causes bleeding, and obscures the colposcopic findings. The technique of forced coughing compared with local anesthesia was evaluated in an RCT of 68 women.[28] Women in the local anesthesia arm received 0.5 mL of 1% lidocaine using a 27-gauge needle. The study was powered to detect a 2-cm difference between the 2 groups on a 0-to 10-cm visual analog scale. There was no difference in mean pain score with cervical biopsy between the 2 groups (lidocaine 1.5, forced coughing 1.9, $P = .47$). However, the time needed for the local anesthesia prolonged the procedure by a median of 2.11 minutes ($P<.001$).

The nonpharmacologic technique of listening to music during colposcopy was investigated in an RCT of 220 women in China where more than 80% of the women received a biopsy.[29] The participants were allowed to choose music from a compilation and it was played over a speaker. The women in the music group experienced significantly less pain (mean 3.32 vs 5.03, $P<.001$) during colposcopic examination than women in the no-music group and had reduced anxiety levels. Music is an easy intervention to implement in the office, via in-office sound systems or through headphones on a patient's own mobile device.

Most effective methods of pain relief for colposcopy and cervical biopsy

- Intracervical injection of local anesthetic
- Forced coughing
- Music

Cervical Dilation and Uterine Aspiration

Dilation of the cervix and uterine aspiration (also known as suction dilation and curettage) with either manual or electric suction is used for induced abortion and the surgical treatment of missed and incomplete abortions. Because many offices do not have electric suction machines, the manual vacuum aspiration (MVA) device enables providers to offer induced abortion or treatment of early pregnancy failures in the office instead of the operating room.[30] This has advantages with regard to patient convenience and no waiting for operating room availability.[31] There was speculation that MVA would be less painful than electric vacuum aspiration because it is quieter but randomized prospective studies demonstrate that there is no difference in the pain experienced.[32] Most women having uterine aspiration procedures in an outpatient setting choose between local anesthesia plus moderate sedation or local anesthesia (paracervical block) with an NSAID with or without an anxiolytic.[33] Although the routine use of misoprostol for cervical ripening before first-trimester uterine aspiration to facilitate dilation and reduce complications remains debated, there is no evidence that misoprostol reduces the pain experienced during the procedure.[34]

Paracervical block

The paracervical block is routinely used for pain management with uterine aspiration procedures performed on awake or moderately sedated patients. The paracervical block is an attempt to anesthetize the nerve bundles lateral to the cervix at 3 o'clock and 9 o'clock as well as those within the uterosacral ligaments. Most experts agree that the paracervical block reduces pain with cervical manipulation and cervical dilation.[1] There is less effect on uterine pain, however. On average, women receiving paracervical block alone with NSAIDs report experiencing moderate pain, ranging from 5 to 7 on a 10-point scale.[35–37] A recent systematic review of paracervical block for surgical abortion showed a lack of documented efficacy with most studies using active treatment arms rather than sham arms for comparison.[38] Nevertheless, in the active treatment arm studies, certain paracervical block techniques were associated with decreased pain such as carbonated lidocaine, deep injection to 3 cm, a 4-site injection, slow injection (over 60 seconds), and waiting 3 minutes between block and dilation.[12] In response to this, Renner and colleagues[12] performed an RCT comparing a paracervical block of 20 mL of 1% buffered lidocaine with 2 mL injected at the tenaculum site followed by injections at 2, 4, 8, and 10 o'clock at the cervicovaginal junction and a sham paracervical block with 2 mL of buffered 1% lidocaine injected at the tenaculum site and no further injections (**Fig. 3**). The injections were deep (3 cm) and 3 minutes were allowed to elapse before dilation. One hundred and twenty women were enrolled, half at less than 8 weeks' gestation and half between 8 and 11 weeks' gestation. Women receiving the paracervical block reported significantly less pain with both dilation (42 vs 79, $P<.001$) and aspiration (63 vs 89, $P<.001$) than women in the sham group. However, women in the paracervical block group reported more pain with the administration of the paracervical block than the sham group (54 vs 30, $P<.001$). These findings were similar for both early and late gestational ages.

Oral medications

NSAIDs Several different NSAIDs have been found to decrease patient-reported pain during uterine aspiration. A study by Wiebe and Rawling[39] found that ibuprofen 600 mg, given 30 minutes preoperatively, improved pain control with aspiration and postoperatively compared with placebo. However, the difference was modest: mean pain with aspiration was 5.07 in the ibuprofen group versus 5.85 in the placebo group, using a scale from 0 to 10. All women were in the first trimester, but average gestational age was higher in the active ibuprofen group (8 vs 6 weeks). In 1984,

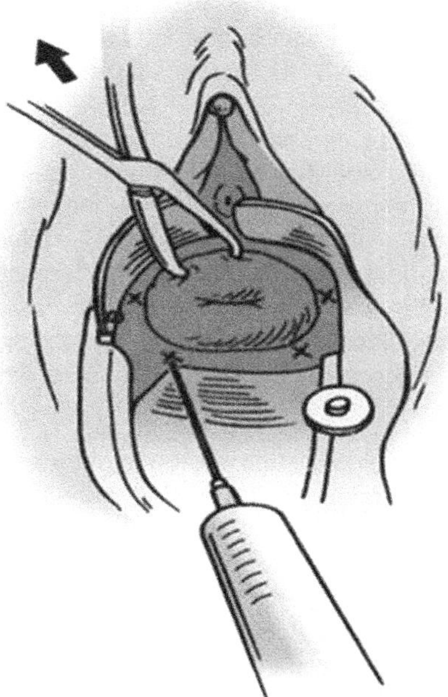

Fig. 3. Paracervical block. (*From* Pfenninger JL, Fowler GC. Pfenninger and Fowler's procedures for primary care. 3rd edition. Philadelphia: Mosby; 2011; with permission.)

Suprapto and Reed[40] concluded that oral naproxen sodium 550 mg given 1 to 2 hours preoperatively significantly decreased intraoperative and postoperative pain. However, a more recent RCT evaluating ketorolac given before surgical abortions under general anesthesia found no difference in postoperative pain.[41] An RCT by Li and colleagues[42] compared misoprostol alone versus misoprostol combined with diclofenac for women having abortions between 7 and 12 weeks' gestation. They found a marginal decrease in pain during the procedure among multiparous subjects only (mean 58 vs 63, P = .06, median 51 vs 68). NSAIDs have not been shown to interfere with the action of exogenous prostaglandins such as misoprostol.

Opioid analgesics A recent placebo-controlled randomized trial evaluated oral hydrocodone-acetaminophen (10 mg/650 mg) among women undergoing first-trimester surgical abortion.[21] All patients received ibuprofen, lorazepam 2 mg, and a paracervical block in addition to hydrocodone-acetaminophen or placebo. There was no difference in visual analog scale pain scores during uterine aspiration (the primary outcome), or at any procedural time point or postoperatively. Pain during uterine aspiration was 63.2 mm for the placebo group and 65.7 mm for the hydrocodone-acetaminophen group (P = .59). However, women in the active hydrocodone-acetaminophen group experienced greater postoperative nausea.

One RCT compared an oral centrally acting analgesic (and weak opioid agonist), tramadol 50 mg, to ibuprofen 800 mg in women undergoing uterine aspiration at less than 20 weeks' gestation.[37] Both were administered 1 hour preoperatively. All women also received a paracervical block and were offered nitrous oxide. They found no difference in immediate postoperative pain, but after 30 minutes, pain scores were significantly lower in the ibuprofen group (2.8 vs 3.6 on a 0 to 10 scale). In another RCT, oral oxycodone 10 mg and sublingual lorazepam 1 mg was compared with an IV regimen with fentanyl 100 μg and midazolam 2 mg.[43] The patients in the IV group had significantly lower intraoperative pain scores on a 0- to 100-mm visual analog scale (61.2 vs 36.3, mean difference 24.9, 95% confidence interval [CI] 15.9–33.9). Pain scores of women in the oral oxycodone arm were comparable with published results for local anesthesia and NSAIDs, suggesting that the oral opioid is no better than local anesthesia alone.

Oral opioids have not been well studied in other gynecologic settings. In 2011, a systematic review and meta-analysis of pain management for office gynecologic procedures (hysteroscopy, hysterosalpingography, sonohysterography, and endometrial ablation) identified only 1 placebo-controlled RCT evaluating an opioid medication.[44] This study of sublingual buprenorphine for hysteroscopy concluded that this medication did not decrease pain but substantially increased side effects including nausea, vomiting, and drowsiness.[45] In summary, there is substantial evidence that opioids are ineffective for decreasing pain with uterine aspiration. They may increase nausea and other adverse effects.

Benzodiazepines Benzodiazepines, such as lorazepam, are anxiolytic medications that have been shown to be safe during first-trimester uterine aspiration.[35,36] However, there are no data suggesting this type of oral medication decreases procedural pain for any gynecologic procedure. In a study of women who self-selected their type of anesthesia, sublingual lorazepam 0.5 to 1 mg did not decrease pain compared with local anesthesia alone and was associated with more dissatisfaction with pain control.[35] A second trial of oral lorazepam given 1 hour preoperatively did not show decreased pain or anxiety.[36] Despite this lack of benefit, in a large survey of members of the National Abortion Federation (NAF), 30% of providers reported offering it at a dose of 1 to 2 mg for first-trimester uterine aspiration.[33]

IV sedation

In 2002, only 21% of National Abortion Federation member clinics offered deep IV sedation or general anesthesia, whereas 33% offered local anesthesia with moderate IV sedation and 46% offered local only with or without oral sedation.[33] For offices with the capacity to offer moderate IV sedation, the doses most often used are 100 μg of fentanyl and 2 mg of midazolam. One study comparing oral and IV sedation with this regimen found that pain scores were 36.3 on a 0- to 100-mm visual analog scale in the IV group compared with 61.2 in the oral group.[43] Using lower doses or only 1 agent is associated with inferior pain control. One randomized trial of 368 women comparing local anesthesia alone to local anesthesia with the addition of intravenous fentanyl (50–100 μg) found that IV fentanyl reduced the pain of first-trimester abortion by only 1.0 point on a 0 to 10 point verbal rating scale, from 5.3 to 4.3.[46] This pain reduction was less than what study participants desired (2.0 points), and the investigators concluded that the pain reduction provided by intravenous fentanyl was of questionable clinical significance. Another randomized study of 100 participants compared local anesthesia alone to local anesthesia in combination with intravenous fentanyl and midazolam.[47] Patients randomized to the treatment arm received 25 μg of fentanyl and 2 mg of midazolam. The treatment arm reported a mean score of 5.5 whereas those in the placebo arm reported a mean score of 5.0, which was not significantly different. However, women who received intravenous sedation reported increased satisfaction with their abortion procedure.

IUD Insertion

The IUD is a long-acting reversible method of contraception that is increasing in popularity in the United States. Approximately 7.7% of women using contraception in the United States use IUDs.[48] The IUD is safe, effective, and has high satisfaction and continuation rates.[49,50] The IUD is now considered appropriate for all women including nulliparous women and adolescents.[51] One barrier to IUDs for contraception is the fear of pain during insertion.[52] Of the IUDs available in the United States, the diameter of the inserter is 3.75 mm for Skyla (Bayer HealthCare Pharmaceuticals Inc, Wayne, NJ, USA), 4.0 mm for Paragard (Teva Women's Health, Inc, Sellersville, PA, USA), and 4.75 mm for Mirena (Bayer HealthCare Pharmaceuticals Inc, Wayne, NJ, USA). Components of the insertion procedure that may cause pain include the tenaculum applied to the cervix to straighten the cervical canal and passing the uterine sound and IUD inserter tube through the internal os of the cervix. Immediately after placement, the IUD may stimulate myometrial contractions causing pain.[53] Factors associated with pain during IUD insertion include nulliparity, lengthier time since last pregnancy or last menses, history of dysmenorrhea, anticipated pain, and not currently breastfeeding. Some, but not all studies, have shown that there is increased pain with levonorgestrel intrauterine system insertion (compared with copper IUD) and older age.[54–59] Studies have shown that up to 21.3% of nulliparous women report severe pain during IUD insertion, and nulliparous women report greater pain during IUD insertion than multiparous women.[54,55,59]

Studies of NSAIDs for pain during IUD insertion have been disappointing. A Danish RCT of 55 women (only 3 nulliparas) found that the median pain level (on a scale of 0 to 10) was 3.[60] Administration of 600 mg of ibuprofen taken 1 to 4 hours before IUD insertion failed to reduce pain compared with placebo during insertion and provided no relief for the following 4 to 6 hours. A randomized placebo-controlled trial of 102 nulliparous and 1916 multiparous women in Chile found that 400 mg of ibuprofen given at least 45 minutes before insertion did not reduce pain in either group.[55] One criticism of these 2 studies is that the ibuprofen dose may have been suboptimal; an effect may have been observed with a dose of 800 mg. However, the 800-mg dose was evaluated in a placebo-controlled RCT of 81, mostly multiparous, women.[61] Ibuprofen 800 mg was given 45 minutes before IUD insertion. Mean pain score on a 10-cm visual analog scale in the placebo group was 3.34 (standard deviation [SD] 2.7) compared with 3.69 (SD 3.4) in the ibuprofen group ($P = .91$). It is unknown whether 800 mg of ibuprofen would have more benefit in certain subgroups, such as nulliparous women, or if taken earlier before insertion such as 1 to 2 hours before the procedure.

Topical 2% lidocaine gel on the cervix is another option that has been used for pain control with IUD insertion. This is used in the United Kingdom but has not been adopted widely in the United States.[62,63] One early trial in 1996 showed decreased pain with 6 mL of 2% lidocaine gel, however, that study lacked proper blinding and allocation concealment.[7,63] Because lidocaine gel does not require an injection, it may be preferable to a paracervical block, which can be painful to administer. However, 2 more recent randomized placebo-controlled trials have failed to find that 2% lidocaine gel applied to the cervix decreased pain with IUD insertion. The first trial of 200 women (30% nulliparous) used 1 mL of gel applied to the internal os of the cervix with a cotton swab for 1 minute.[58] Pain with IUD insertion on a 100-mm visual analog scale was 50.9[32] in the placebo group and 51[31] in the lidocaine group ($P = .98$). In the second trial, all patients received 800 mg of ibuprofen and 0.5 to 1 mL of gel on the anterior lip of the cervix as well as 2 to 3 mL of gel at the internal os for 3 minutes.[17] The investigators enrolled 200 women and randomization was stratified by parity so that there were equal numbers of parous and nulliparous women. Pain scores on a 10-point visual analog scale among the lidocaine and placebo arms were similar for both tenaculum placement (4 vs 4, $P = .15$) and IUD insertion (5 vs 6, $P = .16$) and there was no benefit even among nulliparous women.

Another method of administering local anesthesia, the paracervical block, has been studied in 1 RCT of 50 women receiving IUDs. The study was powered to detect a 20-mm difference in mean pain scores using the 0- to 100-mm visual analog scale. Participants were randomized to receive 2 mL of 1% lidocaine at the tenaculum site and a 10-mL 1% lidocaine paracervical block divided between 8 o'clock and 4 o'clock at the cervical-vaginal junction or no anesthesia. The mean pain score in the lidocaine group at tenaculum placement was 18.8 compared with 29 with no anesthesia ($P = .008$). Mean pain experienced at placement of the paracervical block was 44.7. Nevertheless, mean pain at IUD insertion in the lidocaine group was 37.3 compared with 52.5 in the group with no anesthesia ($P = .09$). The investigators concluded that, using only 10 mL of 1% lidocaine, paracervical block was not effective in reducing IUD insertion pain.[23] However, there was a small effect on reducing pain and it is conceivable that a larger volume block with 20 mL of 1% lidocaine would have a greater effect.

Misoprostol is an effective cervical priming agent before surgical abortion and hysteroscopy and may be helpful in IUD insertions that have proved difficult. Nevertheless, there is no evidence that misoprostol reduces pain with IUD insertion, and it may even increase discomfort with the procedure. One RCT of 80 women demonstrated that 400 μg of sublingual misoprostol administered 1 hour before insertion significantly facilitated IUD placement in nulliparous women but there was no effect on pain.[64] Another trial of 35 nulliparous women randomized to receive 400 μg of buccal misoprostol or placebo 90 minutes before IUD insertion showed no difference on pain between the 2 groups.[65] Moreover, the misoprostol group reported more pre-insertion nausea (29% vs 5%, $P = .05$) and cramping (47% vs 16%, $P = .04$) than the placebo group. A third trial evaluated 400 μg of vaginal misoprostol or placebo 3 hours before IUD insertion among 199 participants, about half of whom were nulliparous.[66]

There was no difference between the 2 groups in pain during insertion or difficulty of insertion as rated by the provider. There were, however, more side effects in the misoprostol arm, predominantly abdominal cramping (44.4% vs 31.5%, $P = .07$). Misoprostol may be useful for women at risk for a difficult insertion such as known cervical stenosis and those who have failed an IUD insertion in the past. However, cervical ripening is not required for all women undergoing IUD insertion and may cause more harm than good. A different cervical ripening agent, nitroprusside (a nitric oxide donor), was studied before IUD insertion in 24 nulliparous women, and was ineffective for decreasing pain or increasing the ease of insertion for providers.[67]

Interventions that do not work for IUD insertion pain

- 2% topical lidocaine gel
- 400 mg, 600 mg, or 800 mg of ibuprofen
- Misoprostol
- Nitroprusside

Office Endometrial Biopsy

Endometrial biopsy (EMB) is 1 of the most commonly performed office gynecologic procedures. When used to evaluate women with abnormal uterine bleeding, EMB has been shown to be as effective as dilation and curettage for diagnosing endometrial pathology such as hyperplasia or malignancy.[68,69] The procedure is generally accomplished with a Pipelle or Explora curette (CooperSurgical, Trumball, CT, USA), which cause a similar degree of pain.[70] The procedure is brief, with the aspiration portion of the biopsy completed within 1 to 2 minutes, but most patients report uncomfortable uterine cramping.

Several studies have evaluated techniques to reduce the discomfort associated with EMB, including topical anesthesia, paracervical block, and intrauterine anesthetic infusions. A randomized study of 20% benzocaine spray applied to the outside of the cervix and into the endocervical canal did not show any benefit compared with placebo among 88 women.[71] Pain scores were 7.5 out of 10 in the intervention group and 8.0 out of 10 in the control group ($P = .61$). According to a recent systematic review by Mercier and Zerden,[72] intrauterine anesthesia seems to be the most effective technique with minimal side effects. The anesthetic does not affect pathologists' interpretation of endometrial samples. Various agents, doses, and infusion techniques have been evaluated for this purpose, and no comparative studies have been published.

Intrauterine instillation can be accomplished with an 18-gauge angiocatheter, Explora curette, metal Novak curette, or other small catheter that can be attached to a syringe. In general, the uterus does not accommodate a large volume of fluid. Most studies have evaluated slow infusion of small quantities (5 mL or less) of more concentrated anesthetic agents (eg, 2% lidocaine), which may serve to minimize cramping and decrease systemic absorption and risk of adverse effects.

In a study by Kosus and colleagues[73] in 2012, women undergoing endometrial biopsy were randomized to receive either paracervical block with 5 mL of 2% lidocaine injected superficially (0.5–1 cm) at 4° and 8 o'clock, intrauterine anesthesia with 5 mL of levobupivacaine, or no intervention. Pain scores among women in the active arms (paracervical block and intrauterine anesthesia) were similar. Both active groups had significantly lower pain scores than those in the placebo group. The study also noted that biopsy indication was a significant predictor of pain, with postmenopausal women experiencing greater pain than premenopausal women with heavy menstrual bleeding. Cicinelli and colleagues[74] evaluated 2 mL of 2% mepivacaine or normal saline infusion before hysteroscopy or office EMB, with a 5-min wait between anesthetic infusion and the procedure. The saline (placebo) group was found to have significantly increased pain as well as a higher incidence of vasovagal reactions. Similarly, Trolice and colleagues[75] randomized 41 women to either 5 mL of 2% lidocaine or saline intrauterine infusion, with a 3-min wait before the procedure. Median pain scores on a 20-cm visual analog scale were 9.9 cm in the placebo group, versus 4.7 cm in the lidocaine group ($P<.01$). In contrast, a trial by Dogan and colleagues[76] randomized 120 women to receive naproxen 550 mg or placebo, along with 5 mL of either 2% intrauterine lidocaine or placebo (4 study groups). Women who received either active naproxen or intrauterine lidocaine had pain scores similar to the placebo group. Only those who received both naproxen and lidocaine reported significantly less pain.

Misoprostol has also been studied as a technique to decrease pain with office endometrial biopsy. Echoing trials of this medication before IUD insertion, misoprostol has not been shown to decrease pain with endometrial biopsy. In a placebo-controlled RCT by Crane and colleagues,[77] 72 women received either oral misoprostol 400 μg or placebo. Women (premenopausal or postmenopausal) in both groups had similar pain (5.8 vs 5.5 cm on the 10-cm visual analog scale, $P = .77$), but those in the misoprostol group more frequently experienced nausea, diarrhea, abdominal pain, cramping, and vaginal bleeding. In a study by Perrone and colleagues,[78] 42 women were randomized to misoprostol 400 μg orally or placebo. Women in the misoprostol group were noted to have significantly more procedural pain ($P<.01$), but there were no differences found in ease of procedure, rate of successful biopsy, cervical resistance, or adverse effects.

Administration of intrauterine anesthesia for endometrial biopsy using Explora or a 5-cm, 18-gauge angiocatheter

- Placement of speculum, cleanse cervix
- Remove Explora stylet, or needle from angiocatheter, and attach syringe with 5 mL of 2% lidocaine
- Insert Explora or angiocatheter to fundus, pull back slightly
- Inject lidocaine slowly (over 1 minute)
- Leave catheter in place for 3 to 5 minutes to minimize backflow

Diagnostic Hysteroscopy

Diagnostic hysteroscopy is frequently performed in the office setting for the evaluation of abnormal uterine bleeding and infertility. The hysteroscope used can be flexible, 3.5 mm outer diameter, or rigid, 3.5 mm outer diameter (minihysteroscope) or 5 mm outer diameter. Pain may prevent the hysteroscopy from being successfully completed in the office setting. The pain during hysteroscopy can come from the speculum placed (if used), the tenaculum placed (if used), the passage of the hysteroscope through the cervix, and the distension of the uterus with fluid. Patients may experience greater pain if other procedures are performed, such as endometrial biopsy, polypectomy, or ablation. In 1 study of 1144 consecutive women who underwent diagnostic hysteroscopy with a 5-mm rigid hysteroscope, carbon dioxide as the distention medium, and endometrial biopsy as indicated, the mean pain score was 4.7 (SD 2.5), and 398 patients (34.8%) experienced severe pain.[79] No local anesthesia or systemic analgesics were used and the surgeons were all experienced. Contrary to what has been noted in most studies of transcervical procedures, they did not find a difference in pain scores between premenopausal and postmenopausal women and nulliparous and multiparous women.

Paracervical block with local anesthesia is an effective technique to reduce pain during office diagnostic hysteroscopy. A recent systematic review showed a benefit to intracervical and paracervical injectable local anesthetic over topical and intrauterine local anesthetics.[80] The investigators were unable to perform analyses in subgroups such as postmenopausal and nulliparous women because of small numbers. Another systematic review confirmed the efficacy of local anesthetics for diagnostic hysteroscopy.[44] They also did not find any evidence to support the use of NSAIDs or oral opioids for outpatient hysteroscopy.

Other techniques to decrease pain during outpatient diagnostic hysteroscopy have been explored. Using normal saline as the distension medium has been shown to be more comfortable for patients compared with carbon dioxide.[81] Warming the distension fluid to 37.5 C compared with room temperature has not been found to reduce pain. An RCT of 67 women using the vaginoscopic approach showed that the mean pain score in the warm fluid group was 3.84 compared with 4.31 in the room temperature fluid group (P = .51).[82] The vaginoscopic approach, performing hysteroscopy without a speculum or tenaculum, causes less pain than traditional hysteroscopy.[6] One trial randomized 126 women to vaginoscopy without anesthesia and the traditional approach with speculum, tenaculum, and 10 mL of 3% mepivacaine intracervical block.[83] The hysteroscopy was performed with normal saline and a rigid 3.7-mm hysteroscope. The women in the vaginoscopy group had mean pain scores of 3.8 compared with 5.3 in the traditional group. Furthermore, the outer diameter of the hysteroscope influences the pain experienced as the instrument is passed through the internal os of the cervix. Trials comparing the traditional 5-mm rigid hysteroscope to the 3.5-mm rigid minihysteroscopes consistently show decreased pain with the smaller diameter instrument.[6] In 1 trial, 6017 procedures with a minihysteroscope were compared with 4204 with a 5-mm hysteroscope.[84] All procedures were performed with the vaginoscopic technique using normal saline and pain was measured on a scale of 0 to 3. In the minihysteroscope group, rates of successful introduction of the scope into the uterine cavity and satisfactory examinations were higher than the 5-mm hysteroscope group (99.5% vs 72.5%, P = <.001% and 98.5% vs 92.3%, P<.001). The mean pain score in the minihysteroscope group was 0.10 (SD 0.34) compared with 1.1 (SD 0.53) in the traditional group (P<.001). In addition, vagal reactions were more common in the traditional group (2.8% vs 0.17%, P<.001).

Hysteroscopic Sterilization

The advent of hysteroscopic tubal occlusion techniques has allowed female sterilization to move from the operating room to the office setting. Hysteroscopic sterilization is less invasive than traditional laparoscopic techniques, presumably leading to a lower risk of serious complications, and is easy to perform.[85] The Essure Permanent Birth Control System (Conceptus Inc, San Carlos, CA) was released in 2002 in the United States. In the Essure procedure, a microinsert containing an inner coil of stainless steel and polyethylene terephthalate (PET) fibers and an outer coil of nickel-titanium is placed in the proximal fallopian tubes under hysteroscopic guidance.[86] The Essure device is compatible with a 5-mm rigid hysteroscope. The manipulation of the fallopian tube may cause additional pain compared with diagnostic hysteroscopy only.

In general, hysteroscopic sterilization is well tolerated in the office. Most providers administer some form of NSAIDs before the procedure to prevent tubal spasm. Among

209 women undergoing hysteroscopic sterilization in the office in the United States, the mean pain score reported was 2.6 (SD 2.05) on a scale of 0 to 10.[87] All women received 60 mg of ketorolac intramuscularly and a 1% lidocaine paracervical block but the amount of lidocaine used was not reported. More than 70% of the women thought that the pain experienced was equal to or less than their menstrual period pain. In a study of 1630 Spanish women, 86.5% of women had minimal to no pain, 10.2% had pain similar to normal menstruation, and only 3.1% felt more pain than with menstruation.[88] The procedures were conducted 1 hour after giving 600 mg of ibuprofen and 10 mg of a benzodiazepine. However, the most painful part of the procedure is placement of the microinserts into the fallopian tubes.[89] There are only 2 RCTs evaluating pain control during hysteroscopic sterilization in the office. In 1 study, 80 women were randomized to a paracervical block of 11 mL of 1% lidocaine or 11 mL of saline.[90] A tenaculum was used after infiltrating 1 mL of lidocaine or saline in the anterior lip of the cervix and 10 mL of lidocaine or saline were used at 4 o'clock and 8 o'clock for a paracervical block. Three to 5 minutes were allowed to elapse before introduction of the hysteroscope. Pain was measured with a 10-cm visual analog scale. Although there was no significant difference in pain with placement of the microinserts into the fallopian tube, the lidocaine group did experience less pain with tenaculum placement (1.0 vs 3.0, $P<.01$), passage of the hysteroscope through the external os (1.5 vs 3.8, $P<.01$), and passage of the hysteroscope through the internal os (1.8 vs 4.1, $P<.01$).

Another double-blind, placebo-controlled study randomized 87 women to intravenous moderate sedation with 2 μg/kg of fentanyl and 2 mg of midazolam or oral analgesia with oxycodone 5 mg and naproxen sodium 500 mg administered 1 hour before the procedure.[91] The goal of the study was to test the equivalence of these medications in the hope that IV placement and IV sedation could be avoided. All participants received 8 mL of 1% lidocaine divided between 4 o'clock and 8 o'clock at the cervix. Pain was measured on a 0- to 100-mm visual analog scale. There were no significant differences between the groups in total pain score or individual scores at speculum insertion, cervical injection of lidocaine, insertion of the hysteroscope, and placement of the first device. Intravenous sedation did lower pain scores at the time of insertion at the second insert compared with oral analgesia. A Cochrane review concluded that paracervical block is a reasonable option for the pain of cervical manipulation during hysteroscopic sterilization because it is safe and inexpensive.[89] However, the ideal regimen for pain control in the office during this procedure has not yet been elucidated.

SUMMARY

The pain experienced from gynecologic procedures is complicated and can be due to not only the physical pain experienced but also the emotional and social factors. No one approach has been discovered that provides the optimal balance of safety and pain control for all women for every type of outpatient gynecologic procedure. However, growing evidence demonstrates that some pain control measures work better than others. Preparing patients for what to expect, understanding their unique needs for pain control, and having a range of options available will allow providers to move some procedures from the operating room to the office.

REFERENCES

1. Nichols MD, Halvorson-Boyd G, Goldstein R, et al. Pain management. In: Paul M, Lichtenberg ES, Borgatta L, et al, editors. Management of unintended and abnormal pregnancy. Hoboken (NJ): Wiley-Blackwell; 2009. p. 90–110.

2. Smith GM, Stubblefield PG, Chirchirillo L, et al. Pain of first-trimester abortion: its quantification and relations with other variables. Am J Obstet Gynecol 1979; 133(5):489–98.
3. Pud D, Amit A. Anxiety as a predictor of pain magnitude following termination of first-trimester pregnancy. Pain Med 2005;6(2):143–8.
4. Belanger E, Melzack R, Lauzon P. Pain of first-trimester abortion: a study of psychosocial and medical predictors. Pain 1989;36(3):339–50.
5. Borgatta L, Nickinovich D. Pain during early abortion. J Reprod Med 1997;42(5): 287–93.
6. Cicinelli E. Hysteroscopy without anesthesia: review of recent literature. J Minim Invasive Gynecol 2010;17(6):703–8.
7. Allen RH, Bartz D, Grimes DA, et al. Interventions for pain with intrauterine device insertion. Cochrane Database Syst Rev 2009;(3):CD007373.
8. American College of Obstetricians and Gynecologists. Report of the Presidential Task Force on Patient Safety in the Office Setting. Washington, DC: ACOG; 2010.
9. Marjoribanks J, Proctor M, Farquhar C, et al. Nonsteroidal anti-inflammatory drugs for dysmenorrhoea. Cochrane Database Syst Rev 2010;(1):CD001751.
10. Wilson LC, Chen BA, Creinin MD. Low-dose fentanyl and midazolam in outpatient surgical abortion up to 18 weeks of gestation. Contraception 2009;79(2): 122–8.
11. McGee DL. Local and topical anesthesia. In: Roberts JR, Hedges JR, editors. Clinical procedures in emergency medicine. 5th edition. Philadelphia: Saunders; 2010.
12. Renner RM, Nichols MD, Jensen JT, et al. Paracervical block for pain control in first-trimester surgical abortion: a randomized controlled trial. Obstet Gynecol 2012;119(5):1030–7.
13. Cepeda MS, Carr DB, Lau J, et al. Music for pain relief. Cochrane Database Syst Rev 2006;(2):CD004843.
14. Akin MD, Weingand KW, Hengehold DA, et al. Continuous low-level topical heat in the treatment of dysmenorrhea. Obstet Gynecol 2001;97(3):343–9.
15. Liberty G, Gal M, Halevy-Shalem T, et al. Lidocaine-prilocaine (EMLA) cream as analgesia for hysterosalpingography: a prospective, randomized, controlled, double blinded study. Hum Reprod 2007;22(5):1335–9.
16. Rabin JM, Spitzer M, Dwyer AT, et al. Topical anesthesia for gynecologic procedures. Obstet Gynecol 1989;73(6):1040–4.
17. McNicholas CP, Madden T, Zhao Q, et al. Cervical lidocaine for IUD insertional pain: a randomized controlled trial. Am J Obstet Gynecol 2012; 207(5):384.e1–6.
18. Davies A, Richardson RE, O'Connor H, et al. Lignocaine aerosol spray in outpatient hysteroscopy: a randomized double-blind placebo-controlled trial. Fertil Steril 1997;67(6):1019–23.
19. Zullo F, Pellicano M, Stigliano CM, et al. Topical anesthesia for office hysteroscopy. A prospective, randomized study comparing two modalities. J Reprod Med 1999;44(10):865–9.
20. Costello MF, Steigrad S, Collet A. A prospective, randomised, single-blinded, controlled trial comparing two topical anaesthetic modalities for the application of a tenaculum to the cervix. J Obstet Gynaecol 2005;25(8):781–5.
21. Micks EA, Edelman AB, Renner RM, et al. Hydrocodone-acetaminophen for pain control in first-trimester surgical abortion: a randomized controlled trial. Obstet Gynecol 2012;120(5):1060–9.

22. Robinson RD, Casablanca Y, Pagano KE, et al. Intracervical block and pain perception during the performance of a hysterosalpingogram: a randomized controlled trial. Obstet Gynecol 2007;109(1):89–93.
23. Mody SK, Kiley J, Rademaker A, et al. Pain control for intrauterine device insertion: a randomized trial of 1% lidocaine paracervical block. Contraception 2010; 86(6):704–9.
24. Church L, Oliver L, Dobie S, et al. Analgesia for colposcopy: double-masked, randomized comparison of ibuprofen and benzocaine gel. Obstet Gynecol 2001;97(1):5–10.
25. Clifton PA, Shaughnessy AF, Andrews S. Ineffectiveness of topical benzocaine spray during colposcopy. J Fam Pract 1998;46(3):242–6.
26. Wong GC, Li RH, Wong TS, et al. The effect of topical lignocaine gel in pain relief for colposcopic assessment and biopsy: is it useful? BJOG 2008;115(8): 1057–60.
27. Oyama IA, Wakabayashi MT, Frattarelli LC, et al. Local anesthetic reduces the pain of colposcopic biopsies: a randomized trial. Am J Obstet Gynecol 2003; 188(5):1164–5.
28. Schmid BC, Pils S, Heinze G, et al. Forced coughing versus local anesthesia and pain associated with cervical biopsy: a randomized trial. Am J Obstet Gynecol 2008;199(6):641.e1–3.
29. Chan YM, Lee PW, Ng TY, et al. The use of music to reduce anxiety for patients undergoing colposcopy: a randomized trial. Gynecol Oncol 2003;91(1): 213–7.
30. Dalton VK, Harris L, Weisman CS, et al. Patient preferences, satisfaction, and resource use in office evacuation of early pregnancy failure. Obstet Gynecol 2006;108(1):103–10.
31. Harris LH, Dalton VK, Johnson TR. Surgical management of early pregnancy failure: history, politics, and safe, cost-effective care. Am J Obstet Gynecol 2007;196(5):445.e1–5.
32. Singh RH, Ghanem KG, Burke AE, et al. Predictors and perception of pain in women undergoing first trimester surgical abortion. Contraception 2008;78(2): 155–61.
33. O'Connell K, Jones HE, Simon M, et al. First-trimester surgical abortion practices: a survey of National Abortion Federation members. Contraception 2009; 79(5):385–92.
34. Cakir L, Dilbaz B, Caliskan E, et al. Comparison of oral and vaginal misoprostol for cervical ripening before manual vacuum aspiration of first trimester pregnancy under local anesthesia: a randomized placebo-controlled study. Contraception 2005;71(5):337–42.
35. Allen RH, Kumar D, Fitzmaurice G, et al. Pain management of first-trimester surgical abortion: effects of selection of local anesthesia with and without lorazepam or intravenous sedation. Contraception 2006;74(5):407–13.
36. Wiebe E, Podhradsky L, Dijak V. The effect of lorazepam on pain and anxiety in abortion. Contraception 2003;67(3):219–21.
37. Romero I, Turok D, Gilliam M. A randomized trial of tramadol versus ibuprofen as an adjunct to pain control during vacuum aspiration abortion. Contraception 2008;77(1):56–9.
38. Renner RM, Jensen JT, Nichols MD, et al. Pain control in first trimester surgical abortion. Cochrane Database Syst Rev 2009;(2):CD006712.
39. Wiebe ER, Rawling M. Pain control in abortion. Int J Gynaecol Obstet 1995; 50(1):41–6.

40. Suprapto K, Reed S. Naproxen sodium for pain relief in first-trimester abortion. Am J Obstet Gynecol 1984;150(8):1000–1.
41. Roche NE, Li D, James D, et al. The effect of perioperative ketorolac on pain control in pregnancy termination. Contraception 2012;85(3):299–303.
42. Li CF, Wong CY, Chan CP, et al. A study of co-treatment of nonsteroidal anti-inflammatory drugs (NSAIDs) with misoprostol for cervical priming before suction termination of first trimester pregnancy. Contraception 2003;67(2):101–5.
43. Allen RH, Fitzmaurice G, Lifford KL, et al. Oral compared with intravenous sedation for first-trimester surgical abortion: a randomized controlled trial. Obstet Gynecol 2009;113(2 Pt 1):276–83.
44. Ahmad G, Attarbashi S, O'Flynn H, et al. Pain relief in office gynaecology: a systematic review and meta-analysis. Eur J Obstet Gynecol Reprod Biol 2011; 155(1):3–13.
45. Lin YH, Hwang JL, Huang LW, et al. Use of sublingual buprenorphine for pain relief in office hysteroscopy. J Minim Invasive Gynecol 2005;12(4):347–50.
46. Rawling MJ, Wiebe ER. A randomized controlled trial of fentanyl for abortion pain. Am J Obstet Gynecol 2001;185(1):103–7.
47. Wong CY, Ng EH, Ngai SW, et al. A randomized, double blind, placebo-controlled study to investigate the use of conscious sedation in conjunction with paracervical block for reducing pain in termination of first trimester pregnancy by suction evacuation. Hum Reprod 2002;17(5):1222–5.
48. Finer LB, Jerman J, Kavanaugh ML. Changes in use of long-acting contraceptive methods in the United States, 2007-2009. Fertil Steril 2012;98(4):893–7.
49. Peipert JF, Zhao Q, Allsworth JE, et al. Continuation and satisfaction of reversible contraception. Obstet Gynecol 2012;117(5):1105–13.
50. Peipert JF, Madden T, Allsworth JE, et al. Preventing unintended pregnancies by providing no-cost contraception. Obstet Gynecol 2012;120(6):1291–7.
51. American College of Obstetricians and Gynecologists. ACOG Committee Opinion No. 392, December 2007. Intrauterine device and adolescents. Obstet Gynecol 2007;110(6):1493–5.
52. Rubin SE, Winrob I. Urban female family medicine patients' perceptions about intrauterine contraception. J Womens Health (Larchmt) 2010;19:735–40.
53. Goldstuck ND. Pain reduction during and after insertion of an intrauterine contraceptive device. Adv Contracept 1987;3(1):25–36.
54. Brockmeyer A, Kishen M, Webb A. Experience of IUD/IUS insertions and clinical performance in nulliparous women–a pilot study. Eur J Contracept Reprod Health Care 2008;13(3):248–54.
55. Hubacher D, Reyes V, Lillo S, et al. Pain from copper intrauterine device insertion: randomized trial of prophylactic ibuprofen. Am J Obstet Gynecol 2006; 195(5):1272–7.
56. Chi IC, Galich LF, Tauber PF, et al. Severe pain at interval IUD insertion: a case-control analysis of patient risk factors. Contraception 1986;34(5):483–95.
57. Chi IC, Wilkens LR, Champion CB, et al. Insertional pain and other IUD insertion-related rare events for breastfeeding and non-breastfeeding women–a decade's experience in developing countries. Adv Contracept 1989;5(2):101–19.
58. Maguire K, Davis A, Rosario Tejeda L, et al. Intracervical lidocaine gel for intrauterine device insertion: a randomized controlled trial. Contraception 2012; 86(3):214–9.
59. Suhonen S, Haukkamaa M, Jakobsson T, et al. Clinical performance of a levonorgestrel-releasing intrauterine system and oral contraceptives in young nulliparous women: a comparative study. Contraception 2004;69(5):407–12.

60. Jensen HH, Blaabjerg J, Lyndrup J. Prophylactic use of prostaglandin synthesis inhibitors in connection with IUD insertion. Ugeskr Laeger 1998;160(48): 6958–61 [in Danish].
61. Chor J, Bregand-White J, Golobof A, et al. Ibuprofen prophylaxis for levonorgestrel-releasing intrauterine system insertion: a randomized controlled trial. Contraception 2011;85(6):558–62.
62. Hollingworth B. Pain control during insertion of an intrauterine device. Br J Fam Plann 1995;21:103–4.
63. Oloto E, Bromham D, Murty J. Pain and discomfort perception at IUD insertion-effect of short-duration, low-volume, intracervical application of two percent lignocaine gel (Instillagel)-a preliminary study. Br J Fam Plann 1996;22:177–80.
64. Saav I, Aronsson A, Marions L, et al. Cervical priming with sublingual misoprostol prior to insertion of an intrauterine device in nulliparous women: a randomized controlled trial. Hum Reprod 2007;22(10):2647–52.
65. Edelman AB, Schaefer E, Olson A, et al. Effects of prophylactic misoprostol administration prior to intrauterine device insertion in nulliparous women. Contraception 2011;84(3):234–9.
66. Dijkhuizen K, Dekkers OM, Holleboom CA, et al. Vaginal misoprostol prior to insertion of an intrauterine device: an RCT. Hum Reprod 2011;26(2):323–9.
67. Bednarek PH, Micks EA, Edelman AB, et al. The effect of nitroprusside on IUD insertion experience in nulliparous women: a pilot study. Contraception 2013;87: 421–5.
68. Ben-Baruch G, Seidman DS, Schiff E, et al. Outpatient endometrial sampling with the Pipelle curette. Gynecol Obstet Invest 1994;37(4):260–2.
69. Demirkiran F, Yavuz E, Erenel H, et al. Which is the best technique for endometrial sampling? Aspiration (pipelle) versus dilatation and curettage (D&C). Arch Gynecol Obstet 2012;286(5):1277–82.
70. Leclair CM, Zia JK, Doom CM, et al. Pain experienced using two different methods of endometrial biopsy: a randomized controlled trial. Obstet Gynecol 2011;117(3):636–41.
71. Einarsson JI, Henao G, Young AE. Topical analgesia for endometrial biopsy: a randomized controlled trial. Obstet Gynecol 2005;106(1):128–30.
72. Mercier RJ, Zerden ML. Intrauterine anesthesia for gynecologic procedures: a systematic review. Obstet Gynecol 2012;120(3):669–77.
73. Kosus N, Kosus A, Guler A, et al. Transcervical intrauterine levobupivacaine infusion or paracervical block for pain control during endometrial biopsy. Exp Ther Med 2012;3(4):683–8.
74. Cicinelli E, Didonna T, Ambrosi G, et al. Topical anaesthesia for diagnostic hysteroscopy and endometrial biopsy in postmenopausal women: a randomised placebo-controlled double-blind study. Br J Obstet Gynaecol 1997;104(3):316–9.
75. Trolice MP, Fishburne C Jr, McGrady S. Anesthetic efficacy of intrauterine lidocaine for endometrial biopsy: a randomized double-masked trial. Obstet Gynecol 2000;95(3):345–7.
76. Dogan E, Celiloglu M, Sarihan E, et al. Anesthetic effect of intrauterine lidocaine plus naproxen sodium in endometrial biopsy. Obstet Gynecol 2004;103(2): 347–51.
77. Crane JM, Craig C, Dawson L, et al. Randomized trial of oral misoprostol before endometrial biopsy. J Obstet Gynaecol Can 2009;31(11):1054–9.
78. Perrone JF, Caldito G, Mailhes JB, et al. Oral misoprostol before office endometrial biopsy. Obstet Gynecol 2002;99(3):439–44.

79. De Iaco P, Marabini A, Stefanetti M, et al. Acceptability and pain of outpatient hysteroscopy. J Am Assoc Gynecol Laparosc 2000;7(1):71–5.
80. Cooper NA, Khan KS, Clark TJ. Local anaesthesia for pain control during outpatient hysteroscopy: systematic review and meta-analysis. BMJ 2010;340:c1130.
81. Shankar M, Davidson A, Taub N, et al. Randomised comparison of distension media for outpatient hysteroscopy. BJOG 2004;111(1):57–62.
82. Evangelista A, Oliveira MA, Crispi CP, et al. Diagnostic hysteroscopy using liquid distention medium: comparison of pain with warmed saline solution vs room-temperature saline solution. J Minim Invasive Gynecol 2011;18(1):104–7.
83. Sagiv R, Sadan O, Boaz M, et al. A new approach to office hysteroscopy compared with traditional hysteroscopy: a randomized controlled trial. Obstet Gynecol 2006;108(2):387–92.
84. Cicinelli E, Parisi C, Galantino P, et al. Reliability, feasibility, and safety of mini-hysteroscopy with a vaginoscopic approach: experience with 6,000 cases. Fertil Steril 2003;80(1):199–202.
85. Duffy S, Marsh F, Rogerson L, et al. Female sterilisation: a cohort controlled comparative study of ESSURE versus laparoscopic sterilisation. BJOG 2005; 112(11):1522–8.
86. Palmer SN, Greenberg JA. Transcervical sterilization: a comparison of essure(r) permanent birth control system and adiana(r) permanent contraception system. Rev Obstet Gynecol 2009;2(2):84–92.
87. Levie M, Weiss G, Kaiser B, et al. Analysis of pain and satisfaction with office-based hysteroscopic sterilization. Fertil Steril 2010;94(4):1189–94.
88. Arjona JE, Mino M, Cordon J, et al. Satisfaction and tolerance with office hysteroscopic tubal sterilization. Fertil Steril 2008;90(4):1182–6.
89. Kaneshiro B, Grimes DA, Lopez LM. Pain management for tubal sterilization by hysteroscopy. Cochrane Database Syst Rev 2012;(8):CD009251.
90. Chudnoff S, Einstein M, Levie M. Paracervical block efficacy in office hysteroscopic sterilization: a randomized controlled trial. Obstet Gynecol 2010; 115(1):26–34.
91. Thiel JA, Lukwinski A, Kamencic H, et al. Oral analgesia vs intravenous conscious sedation during Essure Micro-Insert sterilization procedure: randomized, double-blind, controlled trial. J Minim Invasive Gynecol 2011;18(1): 108–11.

First-Trimester Surgical Abortion Technique

Nicole Yonke, MD, MPH[a,*], Lawrence M. Leeman, MD, MPH[a,b]

KEYWORDS

- First-trimester abortion • Surgical abortion • Electric vacuum aspiration
- Manual vacuum aspiration

KEY POINTS

- First-trimester aspiration abortion is a safe and common procedure that usually occurs in an outpatient setting.
- Complication rates increase gradually with gestational age.
- Postabortal infection prophylaxis should be given before the procedure, not afterward.
- Cervical preparation with misoprostol or osmotic dilators is recommended after 12 weeks' gestation and in adolescents.
- Manual vacuum aspiration is as effective as electric vacuum aspiration.

INTRODUCTION

Abortion is a safe, common procedure in the United States, with 1.21 million abortions performed in 2008 resulting in less than 0.3% of patients hospitalized with complications.[1] Three out of 10 women will have an abortion by 45 years of age, with 74% of abortions occurring in an outpatient clinic.[1,2] Medication abortions with mifepristone have increased in recent years, but 74% of all first-trimester abortions are aspiration procedures.[3] Although women have a constitutionally protected right to an abortion since *Roe v Wade* in 1973, laws regarding gestational age limits, waiting periods, parental consent for minors, and counseling mandates vary state by state. It is imperative to be familiar and comply with local laws before performing pregnancy termination and to review updates frequently.

Funding Sources: None.
Conflict of Interest: None.
[a] Department of Family and Community Medicine, University of New Mexico, MSC 09 5040, 1 University of New Mexico, Albuquerque, NM 87131, USA; [b] Department of Obstetrics and Gynecology, University of New Mexico, MSC 10 5580, 1 University of New Mexico, Albuquerque, NM 87131, USA
* Corresponding author. Department of Family and Community Medicine, University of New Mexico, MSC 09 5040, 1 University of New Mexico, Albuquerque, NM 87131.
E-mail address: nyonke@salud.unm.edu

Obstet Gynecol Clin N Am 40 (2013) 647–670
http://dx.doi.org/10.1016/j.ogc.2013.08.006 obgyn.theclinics.com
0889-8545/13/$ – see front matter

New data have emerged to support changes in first-trimester abortion practice in regard to antibiotic prophylaxis, cervical ripening, the use of manual vacuum aspiration, and pain management. This article addresses these new recommendations and reviews techniques in performing manual and electric vacuum uterine aspiration procedures before 14 weeks' gestation, including very early abortion (<7 weeks' gestation), technically difficult abortions, management of complications, and postabortal contraception. The information discussed also applies to miscarriage management.

INDICATIONS/CONTRAINDICATIONS

Elective termination of pregnancy or miscarriage management is the indication for manual and electric vacuum aspiration, with electric vacuum aspiration usually the choice in the United States after 10 weeks' gestational age. Acute pelvic infection and hemodynamic instability is a contraindication for outpatient abortion. **Table 1** reviews the indications and contraindications for first-trimester surgical abortion.

TECHNIQUE/PROCEDURE

Preparation

Options counseling and consent

- Screen all women to ensure that pregnancy termination is their own voluntary decision and that they feel settled in their decision.
- Alternatives to abortion should be discussed with patients, including parenting and adoption.
- Provide information regarding the risks and benefits of aspiration versus medication abortion if they are candidates for medication abortion.
- Describe the procedure, possible complications, alternatives, and have patients sign a consent form explaining the procedure and risks.
- Discuss pain management options.
- Review postabortal contraceptive options.

Counseling women seeking abortions is an essential component of abortion care. The abortion provider or trained counselor should address how the woman is feeling with open-ended questions and address any fears. The provider should normalize feelings that patients are experiencing. The chapter on "Informed consent, patient education and counseling" in the *Management of Unintended And Abnormal Pregnancy* textbook is an excellent resource for these topics.[4] Although it is important to counsel

Table 1
Indications and contraindications for first-trimester outpatient surgical abortion

Indications	• Elective termination of pregnancy • Management of spontaneous or incomplete abortion
Contraindications	• Acute pelvic infection • Hemodynamic instability
Relative contraindications	• Inability to tolerate the procedure without deep sedation • Coagulopathy • Uncontrolled hypertension, asthma, hyperthyroidism, and epilepsy[a]

[a] These procedures may be performed in an outpatient facility based on provider experience and judgment.

women regarding their options, one small study found that most women had already decided if they wanted an abortion before making an appointment and were fearful of sharing their emotions because of the concern that counselors would try to dissuade them from having an abortion.[5] However, these women still thought counseling was important because they thought that some women may be uncertain or not have the emotional support needed before making their decision.[5]

Medical history

Obtain a complete medical history before the procedure. The Society of Family Planning's (SFP) clinical guideline, "First-trimester abortion in women with medical conditions," provides direction for providers caring for women with chronic medical diseases.[6] Women with uncontrolled medical conditions may need a referral to their primary care provider for management before the procedure or referred for an inpatient procedure. The risk of providing a procedure in the setting of an uncontrolled medical condition should be weighed against the risk of delaying the procedure because abortion complications increase with gestational age.

Bleeding disorders pose a challenge when performing first-trimester abortions. Women with von Willebrand disease have a slight increased risk of bleeding, and those women with severe von Willebrand disease should have their procedures performed in the hospital.[6] No studies have evaluated the effects of antiplatelet agents on bleeding during abortion. If possible, women should stop using antiplatelet agents 5 days before the procedure. For women on anticoagulation with heparin, low-molecular-weight heparin, or warfarin, the risk of transitioning off of anticoagulation versus continued anticoagulation must be balanced. A small study compared women on anticoagulation with women off of anticoagulation and found that, although anticoagulated women had increased blood loss during the procedure, it was not of clinical importance; there were no significant differences in postprocedure hemoglobin between the groups.[7] However, the study was limited because of the small sample size, and most of the women receiving anticoagulation had subtherapeutic levels of low-molecular-weight heparin or a subtherapeutic international normalized ratio at the time of the procedure. In the authors' practice, they perform uterine aspiration in the first trimester in anticoagulated patients in an outpatient setting.

Preprocedure tests

Table 2 discusses routine testing performed before surgical termination.

Clinical examination, dating, and ultrasound

Accurate estimation of gestational age is essential before performing surgical abortion in order to assess the appropriate amount of dilation and the cannula size needed, to determine if cervical ripening is indicated, and to avoid performing a procedure beyond the competency and training of the provider. A bimanual examination is important to estimate the gestational age based on uterine size and to evaluate uterine position. Dating of the pregnancy can be calculated by a last menstrual period that correlates with the uterine size on bimanual examination or by ultrasound. If the last menstrual period is discordant from the clinical examination, uterine fibroids are present, or if the physical examination is limited by obesity, ultrasound can help to confirm gestational age. Ultrasound can also help identify ectopic pregnancy or uterine anomalies before the procedure. After the procedure, if appropriate products of conception for gestational age are not identified, ultrasound should be performed to assess for retained products or other abnormalities. Intraprocedure ultrasound is frequently used and can assist the provider during difficult dilation to visualize the pathway of the cervix or to assess the uterine cavity when anomalies are present. When

Table 2
Preprocedure testing

Confirm pregnancy	• Confirm pregnancy by urine pregnancy test or ultrasound.
Determine Rh(D) status	• Check Rh(D) antigen status before the procedure. • If Rh(D) negative, offer 50 mcg of anti-D immune globulin at the time of the procedure or within 72 h of uterine aspiration to prevent sensitization. A 300-mcg dose of Rho(D) immune globulin may be given if that is all that is available.
STI screening	• The Centers for Disease Control and Prevention recommends routine chlamydia screening for all women younger than 26 y. • Older women at a high risk for sexually transmitted infections or those that request testing may also be screened. • As long as there is not evidence of cervicitis, testing and the procedure can be performed on the same day.
Anemia screening	• Women with a history of anemia or risk factors can be screened with hemoglobin testing before the procedure. • Significant or symptomatic anemia is considered a relative contraindication to an outpatient abortion depending on the facility.

Abbreviation: STI, sexually transmitted infection.

ultrasound is performed, location of the pregnancy, gestational age, fetal number, and presence of cardiac activity should be documented. In 2002, a survey of the members of the National Abortion Federation found that 92% used ultrasound to confirm gestational age when providing first-trimester abortions.[8] However, data on the benefit of routine ultrasound use during abortion care are limited, with one review finding no evidence of improved safety or efficacy of abortion with the use of preprocedure ultrasound.[9]

TECHNIQUE/PROCEDURE

The procedure equipment is described in **Box 1** and **Fig. 1**.

1. Position the woman in the dorsal lithotomy position, with her feet in stirrups or leg holders. Her hips should be positioned at the end of the table with her buttocks slightly off the edge of the table.
2. Perform a bimanual examination to verify the size and position of the uterus.
3. Place a speculum and visualize the cervix. If there is difficulty visualizing her cervix, a knee-to-chest position may be helpful.
4. If using cervical specimens to screen for gonorrhea or chlamydia, collect a cervical swab.
5. *Optional*: Prepare the vagina and cervix with povidone-iodine or chlorhexidine. The SFP finds no evidence to support this practice over saline to reduce infections but also notes that it is not associated with harm.[10]
6. Place 2 mL of 0.5% or 1.0% lidocaine into the cervix superficially where the tenaculum will be placed.
7. Place the tenaculum. Most providers place the tenaculum on the anterior cervical lip; however, if the uterus is extremely retroflexed, some providers find it useful to the place the tenaculum on the posterior cervical lip. Place at least 1 cm of cervical tissue into the tenaculum in order to have adequate traction that is needed to straighten the cervical canal and to minimize the likelihood of the cervix tearing

Box 1 **Procedure equipment**
Speculum
Atraumatic or singled-toothed tenaculum
22- to 27-g spinal needle or 22- to 27-g needle with 3-in needle extender
0.5% or 1.0% lidocaine with epinephrine, vasopressin, or 8.6% sodium bicarbonate
Cervical dilators
Osmotic dilators (if indicated)
Misoprostol (if indicated preprocedure or available for hemorrhage)
Ring forceps
4 × 4 gauze
Cannula
Manual vacuum aspirator or electronic vacuum aspirator with tubing
Bowl for products of conception
Small sharp curette: size 0, 1, or 2
Mesh strainer
Glass container to view products of conception
Backlight
Povidone-iodine solution
Specimen container for pathology if indicated

during traction. The tenaculum may be placed horizontally or vertically with one side within the cervical canal.

8. Perform a paracervical block (PCB). There are a variety of techniques and anesthetic solutions used for a PCB. A common solution is 0.5% to 1.0% lidocaine with additives of vasopressin or epinephrine for vasoconstriction and the addition of sodium bicarbonate for buffering to decrease pain with injection (**Box 2**).

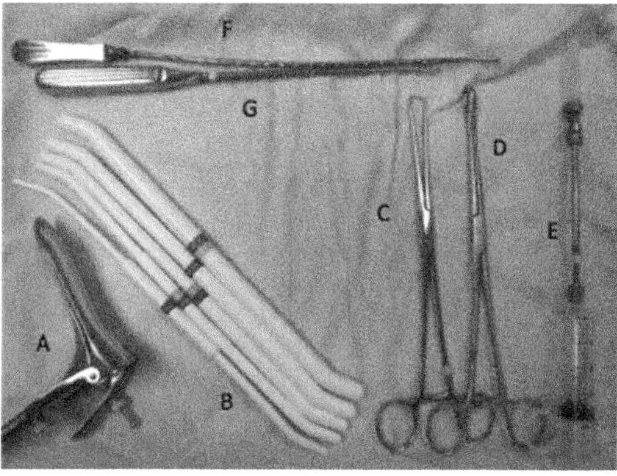

Fig. 1. Uterine aspiration tray. A, speculum; B, Denniston dilators; C, tenaculum; D, ring forceps; E, syringe with needle extender; F, uterine sound; G, curette. (With permission from UNM Center for Reproductive Health, May 2013.)

Box 2
PCB mixture

18 mL 0.5% or 1.0% lidocaine

1.5 units of vasopressin

2 mL of 8.4% sodium bicarbonate

Vasopressin has the advantage of producing less tachycardia and anxiety with administration compared with epinephrine. After the 2 mL is injected into the cervix for tenaculum placement, the additional 18 mL should be injected for the PCB. Injections should be made at the reflection of the cervix with the vaginal mucosa. Including deeper injections into the uterine muscle has been demonstrated to provide improved analgesia compared with only injecting superficially at the junction of cervix and vagina.[11] Some providers inject at 2, 4, 8, and 10 o'clock, whereas other prefer to inject at only 4 and 8 o'clock. The anesthetic solution should be slowly injected while inserting and withdrawing the needle. Aspiration should be performed before injecting to check for vessels and avoid an intravascular injection.

9. Cervical dilation
   a. A modified sterile technique, the no-touch approach, may be used throughout the procedure to maintain the sterility of the uterine cavity whereby the provider does not touch the part of the instruments entering the uterus; the dilators are only touched in the center so that the tips on both sides entering the uterus remain sterile. Alternatively, a full sterile technique may be used.
   b. As a general rule, dilate to the millimeter equal to the gestational age in weeks. For example, dilate to 7 mm for a 7-week gestation.
   c. Starting with a 5-mm Denniston or 17F Pratt, the dilator can be gently inserted into the cervix, holding it like a pencil in the midline, careful to not exert too much force. Sounding the uterus before the procedure is not necessary.
   d. At the same time, steady force on the tenaculum should be used to bring the cervix toward the provider to straighten out the cervical canal and decrease the angle between the cervix and uterus. Some resistance may be noted at the internal os. If the cervix feels tight, the dilator should be left in place for 10 to 20 seconds before advancing to the next size.
   e. Depending on the baseline dilation of the cervix, one may choose to use the next size dilator or skip to a larger dilator if the cervix is already dilated. Continue dilating until the desired cannula size (based on the gestational age) is reached, or stop earlier if the cervix provides too much resistance to continue dilating safely.
   f. If there is initial difficulty with dilation, try slowly twisting the dilator to find the pathway through the cervix. An os finder or uterine sound can also be used. The cervical canal and uterus can also be visualized with ultrasound guidance, allowing direct visualization of the dilator in the cervix. Cervical ripening agents, such as osmotic dilators or misoprostol, can help soften the cervix and ease dilation. For early gestations when dilation is difficult, consider delaying the procedure for cervical preparation or offering a medication abortion.
   g. For obese patients, there may be a relatively longer vaginal vault and excess soft tissue, which may create difficulty reaching the cervix holding the dilators in the midpoint as outlined earlier. A full sterile technique may be used or a second set of dilators may be used to hold each dilator at the end, ensuring a proper no-touch technique but allowing for adequate maneuvering capability.

10. Vacuum aspiration
    a. Keeping the tip sterile, insert the appropriate size of cannula through the os to the uterine cavity. Some providers will advance to the fundus, whereas others prefer to put the cannula only into the cavity to avoid the risk of perforation. Some providers prefer to place the cannula into the uterus and then attach the vacuum aspirator (VA), whereas others insert in the cannula with the VA already attached. If the VA is attached during insertion, be sure that the suction is not on.
        i. Manual vacuum aspiration (MVA): Create a vacuum by closing the valves and pulling back on the plunger. After the cannula is inserted into the uterus, open the valves to create suction.
        ii. Electric vacuum aspiration (EVA): The thumb switch should be closed and the cannula inserted into the uterus. The EVA machine can then be powered on to create suction. Release the thumb valve to stop the suction when removing the cannula from the cervical canal.
        iii. For patients with a tortuous or angulated cervix/uterus: Consider ultrasound guidance to minimize the risk of perforation. If there is difficulty placing the cannula after dilation because of curvature of the cervix/uterus, a sterile sound may be placed and the cannula inserted over the sound. The sound can be removed and the vacuum aspirator attached. Note that sterile gloves must be used because the cannula will pass over the sound.
    b. Aspirate the uterine contents using a twirling or back-and-forth motion, being cautious of where the fundus is located to avoid perforation and excess pain. Aspiration should be continued until the uterus has a sandpaper or gritty sensation that indicates an empty uterus and there is little tissue passing through the cannula. If using an MVA, multiple passes may be necessary because the MVA loses suction as the cylinder fills. This scenario is more common with more advanced gestational ages.
    c. If there is no passage of tissue through the cannula, it may be clogged. Try adjusting it within the uterine cavity to see if flow returns. If not, remove the cannula from the uterus and reinsert it. If using an MVA, check to make sure it is working properly and suction is created when it is loaded. Suction may also be lost with an MVA because of overdilation. A larger cannula may have to be used to create suction in this situation.
11. Evaluate the products of conception (POC): POC evaluation is important to ensure completion of the procedure and decrease the risk of unrecognized ongoing pregnancy. Wash the POC in a mesh strainer to remove the blood and clot. Place the POC in a glass dish and add water or normal saline solution. Place the dish over a backlight. A gestational sac, chorionic villi, blood, decidua, and possibly fetal parts, depending on gestational age, will be seen. Please see **Table 3**, "Gestational age and expected POC" and **Fig. 2**, "POC." The findings should correlate with the expected gestational age. All suspected molar pregnancies, based on ultrasound findings or hydropic chorionic villi on inspection, should be sent to pathology for evaluation. If a procedure was performed without a confirmed intrauterine pregnancy and review of POCs did not definitively identify a gestational sac, then the POCs may be sent to pathology to determine if an intrauterine pregnancy was present and serial human chorionic gonadotropin (hCG) levels should be followed. An ultrasound to evaluate for unsuccessful uterine aspiration or ectopic pregnancy should be performed in this scenario, and the woman should receive standard ectopic precautions. No benefit has been found from routinely

Table 3
Gestational age and expected POC

Gestational Age (wk)	POC
5	Gestational sac ~5 mm
6	Gestational sac ~10 mm, dime size
7	Gestational sac ~15 mm, nickel size
8	Gestational sac ~10 mm, quarter size
9	Small fetal parts + gestational sac, foot length, 4 mm
10	4 extremities, spine, calvarium, gestational sac, foot length, 6 mm
11	4 extremities, spine, calvarium, gestational sac, foot length, 7–8 mm
12	4 extremities, spine, calvarium, gestational sac, placenta, foot length, 9 mm
13	4 extremities, spine, calvarium, gestational sac, placenta, foot length, 11 mm

sending POC for histologic examination in the absence of clinical suspicion of a failed procedure, ectopic pregnancy, or molar pregnancy.[12]

12. Insert an intrauterine contraceptive, if requested, after completion of the abortion is confirmed by reviewing the POC or ultrasound.
13. Remove the tenaculum from the cervix. Evaluate for bleeding. Gently remove blood from the vaginal vault with a sponge stick or large cotton-tipped swab. Remove the speculum.
14. Observe the patient for pain or bleeding for 15 minutes after the procedure. If she had moderate sedation, she should be observed until she is at her baseline mental status, which will vary by patient and may be 1 to 2 hours after the procedure. Please refer to "Practice Guidelines for Sedation and Analgesia by the Non-Anesthesiologist"[13] for recommendations.
15. Discuss the discharge instructions and provide written materials with emergency contact numbers if needed.

ANTIBIOTIC PROPHYLAXIS TO PREVENT POSTPROCEDURAL INFECTIONS

A single preoperative dose of doxycycline up to 12 hours preceding a surgical abortion is recommended to prevent postabortal upper genital tract (UGT) infections.[10]

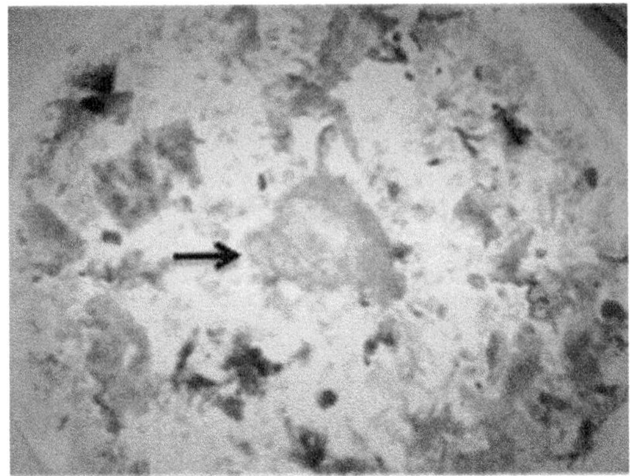

Fig. 2. POC. Gestational sac marked by arrow. (With permission from UNM Center for Reproductive Health, May 2013.)

Although it has been common in the past to initiate antibiotics after the procedure for infection prophylaxis, this has not been demonstrated to be of benefit and is discouraged.[10] Risk factors for postabortal infection are current infection with *Chlamydia trachomatis*, *Neisseria gonorrhoeae*, and bacterial vaginosis. Studies have demonstrated that universal prophylaxis is more cost-effective than screen-and-treat strategies.[10] Prophylactic antibiotic use is associated with a 59% reduction in postabortal UGT infections, although the baseline risk is low, with more than 1 in 100 women needing prophylaxis to prevent one infection.[10,14] Despite the low baseline risk of infection, the benefit of universal prophylaxis outweighs the minimal risks of treatment, including photosensitivity and nausea. Metronidazole can be used as an alternative to doxycycline, but there is less evidence to support its efficacy in preventing infections; routinely using it in addition to doxycycline to treat bacterial vaginosis does not reduce the infection risk.[10]

CERVICAL PREPARATION

Osmotic dilators, such as *Laminaria* (*Laminaria digita* and *Laminaria japonicum*) and synthetic, hygroscopic polyacrylonitrile dilators (Dilapan-S, GelMed International s.r.o., Kamenne Zehrovice, Czech Republic), have been used extensively to prepare the cervix. Recent data suggest misoprostol and mifepristone are effective cervical ripening agents. See **Table 4**, "Osmotic dilators." Evidence regarding the use of

Table 4
Osmotic dilators

Dilator	Description	Onset of Action	Advantages	Disadvantages
Laminaria (*Laminaria digita, Laminaria japonicum*)	Dried stalks of hygroscopic seaweed	• Absorb water from cervical stroma • Swell to 3–4 times dry diameter • Apply pressure to cervical walls and induce prostaglandins to promote dilation • Increases in size by 25% in 4 h and 90% overnight	• Inexpensive • Possible decrease in cervical laceration in older studies	• Acts slowly • Requires second visit • Small risk of hypersensitivity reaction • Small risk of bacterial spore exposure, but no difference in infection incidence
Hygroscopic Polyacrylonitrile (Dilapan-S)	Synthetic made from polyacrylate-based hydrogel Sizes 3 × 55 mm 4 × 55 mm 4 × 65 mm	• Absorb water from cervical tissue • 3-mm swells to 8–9 mm in 4 h • 4-mm swells to 10–11 mm in 4 h	• Rapid swelling • 1-d procedure • Increased swelling compared with *Laminaria* at 4 h, equiva lent at 6 h	• More expensive than *Laminaria*

Data from Allen RH, Goldberg AB, Board of Society of Family Planning. Cervical dilation before first-trimester surgical abortion (<14 weeks' gestation). SFP guideline 20071. Contraception 2007;76(2):139–56.

cervical ripening agents to prevent complications in the first trimester remains mixed, partly because of a very low baseline risk of complications, especially for experienced providers. Cervical injuries are estimated to be 0.1 to 10.0 per 10,000, and clinically apparent uterine perforation ranges from 0.1 to 4.0 per 1000 procedures.[15] The risk of complications is higher for adolescents, regardless of parity, and for increasing gestational ages.[15] Because of this increased risk, the SFP recommends the consideration of cervical priming for adolescents, for all women at 12 to 14 weeks' gestation, and anytime there is initial difficulty with dilation.[15] See **Table 5**, "Guidelines on cervical preparation." A Cochrane review found a shorter procedure time with the use of cervical preparation but no decrease in complications.[16] Most providers use mechanical dilation without cervical preparation for surgical abortions at less than 12 weeks' gestation because complication risks are low and cervical priming requires more time and has side effects. There is little evidence on the effect of cervical priming on procedural pain.

Misoprostol, a prostaglandin E1 synthetic analogue, is the most commonly used medication for cervical priming and has the advantages of low cost and quick onset, allowing 1-day procedures.[15] Misoprostol can be absorbed via oral, buccal, sublingual, vaginal, or rectal routes. The different routes of administration are associated with different absorption times, peak plasma levels, and side effects. Sublingual misoprostol has higher peak serum levels and is more quickly absorbed than other routes of administration, with a similar area under the curve to vaginal administration.[15] Vaginal misoprostol has slower absorption than oral or sublingual but with a greater area under the curve than oral. Buccal absorption has lower serum levels compared with vaginal but a similar onset. Rectal administration has the lowest peak concentration and lowest area under the curve.

The dose of 400 mcg of sublingual misoprostol is effective 2 hours after administration.[17] Multiple studies have evaluated the dosing and timing of vaginal misoprostol. According to the SFP, the optimal dose of misoprostol is 400 mcg; however, the timing before the procedure depends on the route of administration: 3 to 4 hours for vaginal administration, 8 to 12 hours orally, or 2 to 3 hours sublingually.[15] Comparing routes of

Table 5
Guidelines on cervical preparation

Society	Recommendation
World Health Organization[69]	Cervical priming recommended for • Women aged younger than 18 y • Nulliparous women >9 wk gestation • All women >12 wk gestation
Royal College of Obstetricians[70] and Gynecologists	Consider cervical preparation for all procedures, but it is most beneficial when risk factors are present. "Evidence is insufficient to determine at what gestational age cervical priming should be routine."
National Abortion Federation[71]	"Cervical dilation may be facilitated through the use of osmotic dilators or misoprostol, particularly in adolescents or women at risk for cervical stenosis."
Planned Parenthood[72]	Use of cervical priming is optional for first-trimester abortions
SFP[72]	Cervical priming recommended for • Adolescents, especially if gestational age is >12 wk • All women at gestational age >12–14 wk • Any women with initial difficult dilation

administration, sublingual administration is superior to vaginal administration when used 2 to 3 hours before the procedure but may be equivalent at later times and is associated with more nausea, vomiting, and diarrhea.[16,18,19] Vaginal misoprostol results in superior dilation and fewer side effects compared with oral administration 3 hours before a procedure.[20] Buccal administration is less studied; but based on its pharmacologic similarities to vaginal administration, it is effective at 400 mcg given 3 to 4 hours before a procedure.[15,21] See **Table 6**, "Misoprostol for cervical priming." Waiting longer than 3 to 4 hours to perform a procedure after the administration of misoprostol may result in bleeding and passing of POC before the procedure.

A recently published study comparing 125 women between 12 and 15 weeks' gestation receiving 400 mcg of buccal misoprostol or one hygroscopic polyacrylonitrile dilator administered 3 to 4 hours before a procedure found both methods to be equivalent regarding pain with the procedure, procedure time, complications, and satisfaction; however, women receiving misoprostol had more pain associated with cervical ripening.[21] In contrast, a study comparing one medium-sized *Laminaria* and 400 mcg of vaginal misoprostol found equivalent dilation with both regimens, but more pain with cervical ripening was reported in the *Laminaria* group.[22] Both the Cochrane and SFP reviews found misoprostol and osmotic dilators to be equivalent for cervical ripening but that there is little data to support their use for reducing complications in first-trimester procedures.[15,16] One large trial (that was not included in

Table 6
Misoprostol for cervical priming

Route	Regimen	Advantages	Disadvantages
Vaginal	• 400 mcg 3–4 h before procedure • Higher doses did not improve cervical dilation • Lower doses were less effective	• Likely more effective than oral administration	• After 4 h more likely to pass pregnancy before procedure
Buccal	• 400 mcg 3–4 h before procedure	• Similar pharmacokinetics as vaginal • Avoids vaginal administration	• Less data on use
Sublingual	• 400 mcg 2–3 h before procedure • 400 mcg is more effective than 200 mcg but associated with more side effects	• More effective than oral regimen • Equivalent or possibly more effective than vaginal • Quicker onset of action • Avoids vaginal administration	• More GI side effects
Oral	• 400–600 mcg 3–20 h before procedure	• Avoids vaginal administration	• Preferred by staff • Longer onset of action

Abbreviation: GI, gastrointestinal.

Adapted from Allen RH, Goldberg AB, Board of Society of Family Practice. Cervical dilation before first-trimester surgical abortion (<14 weeks' gestation). SFP guideline 20071. Contraception 2007;76(2):139–56.

these reviews) by the World Health Organization of 4970 women did find that less than 1% of multiparous women receiving 400 mcg of misoprostol vaginally required re-evacuation for incomplete abortion compared with 2% of multiparous women receiving placebo (relative risk [RR] 0.08, 95% confidence interval [CI] 0.08–0.44).[23] This finding was not statistically significant for nulliparous women.

PAIN CONTROL

The pharmacologic methods studied to reduce pain during first-trimester abortion are PCB, premedication with oral nonsteroidal antiinflammatory drugs, anxiolytics, opiates, intravenous (IV) mild to moderate sedation, and general anesthesia. The "Practice guidelines for sedation by non-anesthesiologists," from the American Society of Anesthesiologists can be used as a reference for providing IV sedation.[13] The best approach to pain control during first-trimester abortion has not been established, but most women report decreased pain when receiving IV sedation compared with oral medications.[24] Various methods of pain control for surgical abortion are summarized next.

PCB

A Cochrane review published in 2009 found insufficient data to show a benefit of a PCB compared with no block.[25] However, a 2012 study found PCB to reduce pain during first-trimester abortion.[26] In this study, women were premedicated with ibuprofen and lorazepam. Eighteen mL of 1% lidocaine with 2 mL of 8.4% sodium bicarbonate were injected at 2, 4, 8, and 10 o'clock at the cervicovaginal reflection from superficial to 3 cm deep over 60 seconds, injecting with insertion and withdrawal. Dilation was performed 3 minutes after the block. This block significantly decreased pain scores with dilation and aspiration and improved satisfaction with the procedure. In another study, the addition of ketorolac in the PCB demonstrated less pain with dilation, but there was no difference in procedural pain, postprocedural pain, or satisfaction with the procedure.[27]

Oral Medications With PCB

Premedication with ibuprofen and naproxen resulted in a small reduction in pain scores in a Cochrane review.[25] In contrast, hydrocodone and acetaminophen did not result in decreased pain scores or increased patient satisfaction.[28]

IV Sedation

IV benzodiazepines and opioids in addition to PCB was found to significantly reduce pain in a Cochrane review compared with women only receiving a PCB.[25] In studies comparing PCB with oral oxycodone or lorazepam to IV sedation, women reported significantly less pain and greater satisfaction with IV sedation.[24,25,29] Many clinics require fasting before minimal or moderate sedation in order to reduce complications related to anesthesia; however, one retrospective cohort study of not fasting before minimal to moderate sedation in 47,748 women undergoing aspiration abortion found no reports of anesthesia complications, estimating the expected incidence of complications to be 0.00006%.[30]

General Anesthesia

General anesthesia is associated with less intraoperative pain but more postoperative pain compared with moderate sedation.[25] Blood loss was increased with inhalation anesthetics.[25]

Music

Multiple studies have evaluated the effect of music on pain during procedures with mixed results on whether pain was increased, decreased or unchanged.[25,31,32]

MVA, EVA, MECHANICAL DILATION, AND CANNULA

First-trimester surgical abortion is performed by MVA or EVA. In the past, sharp curettage was used without vacuum aspiration; however, this has been associated with more pain, increased risk of perforation, and does not decrease the risk of retained POC.[33]

MVA

An MVA is a 60-mL syringe cylinder that can accommodate multiple cannula sizes with a plunger and valves that create a vacuum of 60 mm Hg when pulling on the plunger, equivalent to an electric vacuum (see **Fig. 3**, "MVA"). Depending on the gestational age of the pregnancy, an MVA may need to be emptied multiple times during a procedure, requiring more passes in the uterus. Although there are no clear gestational age limits for MVA use, most providers will use it up until 8 to 10 weeks' gestation. In the United States, Ipas (Chapel Hill, NC) and MedGyn (Lombard, IL) manufacture MVAs. MVAs can be used one time or may be reused if they are cleaned according to the manufacturer's instructions.

EVA

EVA requires a suction machine with an attached single-use or reusable hose and a rotating handle where different sized cannulas can be attached. EVA is noisier than MVA; however, placing the suction machine in an adjacent room can reduce the noise. EVA requires fewer passes of the uterus because there is no need to reload an aspirator, which can make it easier to remove larger POC and decrease the procedure time.

MVA and EVA are equally effective in successfully completing abortion procedures with similar incidences of complications. Studies find that some women are bothered by the noise of EVA.[33–37] In a Cochrane review, women less than 9 weeks' gestation reported less pain with MVA (RR 0.73, 95% CI 0.47–1.16).[33] Providers perceived more difficulty using MVA compared with EVA after 9 weeks' gestation (RR 5.7, 95% CI 2.45–13.28).[33] One study found a longer procedure time for MVA compared with EVA.[38]

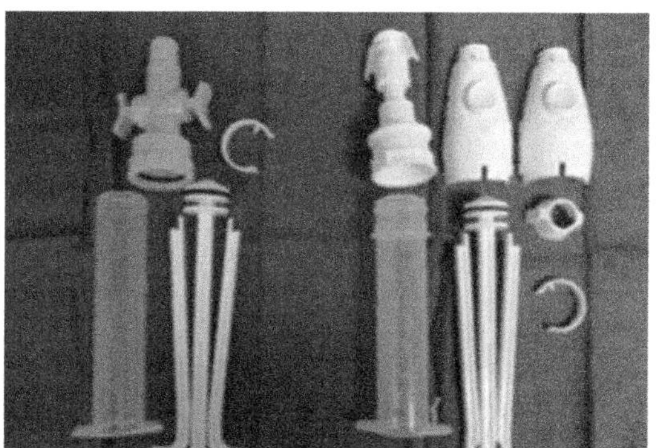

Fig. 3. MVA. (With permission from UNM Center for Reproductive Health, May 2013.)

Cannula

A flexible, rigid straight or rigid curved disposable plastic cannula can be used with both EVA and MVA, depending on provider preference. There is no difference in cervical injury, infection, blood transfusion, incomplete abortion, or need for repeat aspiration between the cannula types.[33] The size of cannula to use for a procedure varies by the provider. Most providers will use a cannula in millimeters equal to the gestational age.[8]

Mechanical Dilators

The SFP recommends using tapered dilators, such as Pratt or Denniston, and advises against the use of blunt dilators, such as Hegar, because they requiring more force with dilation and there is a concern for an increased risk of perforation.[15]

ABORTION BEFORE 7 WEEKS' GESTATION

Abortion at a very early gestational age may be complicated by the inability to confirm an intrauterine pregnancy on ultrasound before the procedure or difficulty identifying a gestational sac on inspection of the tissue after the procedure. The SFP's clinical guidelines state that procedures in women without a confirmed intrauterine pregnancy may still be performed if there are adequate follow-up protocols in place.[39] If a gestational sac is not visualized after aspiration, the woman should have serial serum hCG titers to exclude ectopic pregnancy and ensure resolution of the aspirated pregnancy. The serum hCG should decrease by at least 50% within 48 hours of the procedure.[39] Examination of the POC by a pathologist may confirm an IUP when a gestational sac cannot be seen by visual examination; however, serial quantitative hCG measurements are still indicated in this scenario to ensure a successfully completed abortion. Failed surgical abortion before 7 weeks' gestation is uncommon, varying from 1 to 23 per 1000 aspirations.[39] MVA and EVA are equally efficacious in early pregnancy termination, and there is no difference in the ability to identify the POC after aspiration.[40]

THE DIFFICULT ABORTION

Although first-trimester surgical abortion is usually accomplished easily and without complications, occasionally difficulty will be encountered. Obstacles to abortion include difficulty identifying the cervical os, accomplishing adequate dilation to enter the uterine cavity, or successfully aspirating the pregnancy. Uterine anomalies or ectopic pregnancy location must be considered when difficulties are encountered.

After the speculum is placed, the physician may not be able to see the cervix because of the obscured visualization from vaginal mucosa or because of extreme uterine retroversion or anteversion. Repeating the bimanual examination may assist in locating the cervix. Changing the speculum size or type may provide an improved view. A long Pederson speculum can help visualize a cervix that is deep inside the vagina and the large Graves may be helpful for an obese woman. Sidewall refractors may be used to clear the vaginal mucosa from the provider's view through the speculum. Once the cervix is partially seen a tenaculum can be placed to bring the cervix into fuller view.

In other cases the cervix may be easily seen, but the opening of the cervical os may not be identifiable. This most commonly occurs in women of reproductive age as a result of cervical stenosis that can occur secondary to the use of cryotherapy, loop electrical excision, or cold knife cone biopsy to treat cervical dysplasia.[41] The use of a plastic os finder can facilitate identification of the cervical opening. If the os is too small to place a 5 mm dilator then smaller dilators such as lacrimal duct probes may be used. A plastic endometrial suction curette used for endometrial biopsy can facilitate determining the direction of the endocervical canal and avoid the creation of a false passageway during dilation.

On occasion, there may be appropriate cervical dilation to enter the uterine cavity, but difficulty is encountered with aspiration of the pregnancy tissue. This problem may occur because of a difficult angle of the uterine cervix and cavity, which does not permit the suction curette to reach a fundal pregnancy. Increasing the degree of cervical dilation or using a flexible curette that can bend to reach the gestational sac may alleviate this problem. In these situations, ultrasound guidance may increase the likelihood of successful aspiration and reduce the chance of uterine perforation.

Ultrasound may also be very helpful in the difficult aspiration by permitting the identification of a uterine anomaly.[42] A woman with a bicornuate uterus may have the curette placed in the wrong horn, in which case aspiration will not be successful regardless of how long the procedure is attempted. Once the uterine anatomy is identified, the provider can usually use ultrasound guidance to reach the proper cavity. With a uterine didelphys, whereby there are 2 separate cervix and uteri, the correct cervix must be entered (**Fig. 4**). A metal sound, which can be easily seen on ultrasound, can assist in confirming the appropriate location of the cannula. Ultrasound may also allow for the identification of a pregnancy that is not located in the endometrial cavity of the uterus. At times, a preprocedure ultrasound may identify and measure a crown rump length without noting that the location is outside the uterus. A repeat ultrasound whereby care is taken to identify the uterus will usually allow for the correct diagnosis. A cornual pregnancy can be challenging to diagnosis because the pregnancy is partially within the uterus. The key diagnostic feature on ultrasound of a cornual pregnancy is the inability to identify myometrium circumferentially around the gestational sac. If a cornual pregnancy is suspected, the procedure should not be performed in an outpatient setting. Cervical pregnancy is quite uncommon; however, proper identification is essential because attempts to aspirate a cervical pregnancy can lead to uncontrolled bleeding and management of this type of ectopic pregnancy requires treatment with methotrexate or other modalities (**Fig. 5**).

Whenever surgical abortion is difficult, consideration should be given to the option of medication abortion with mifepristone. Mifepristone is FDA approved up to 49 days estimated gestational age, but is commonly used at higher gestational ages based on

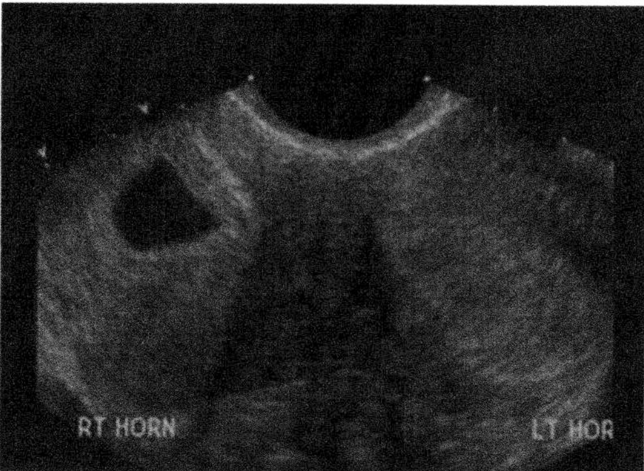

Fig. 4. Bicornuate uterus with pregnancy in right horn. (With permission from Matthew Reeves, mreeves@prochoice.org.)

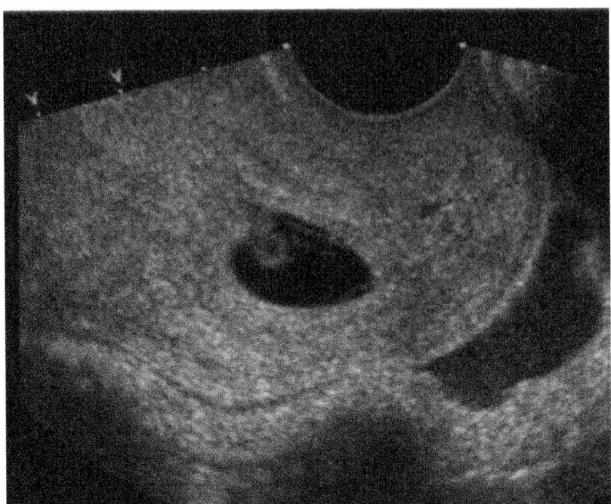

Fig. 5. Cervical ectopic. (With permission from Matthew Reeves, mreeves@prochoice.org.)

studies demonstrating safety and efficacy up to 9 weeks or 63 days when accompanied by vaginal or buccal misoprostol.[43] Recent data support the use of mifepristone for outpatient abortion through 70 days' gestation, demonstrating similar safety and effectiveness as those performed at 9 weeks' gestation.[44] Mifepristone and misoprostol may also be used from 10 to 13 weeks; however, this will require a setting whereby a repeated dose of misoprostol may be used and patients safely observed given the potential for heavier bleeding at this later gestational age. Depending on the regional laws and political realities, this could occur in a labor or delivery or inpatient gynecology unit.

COMPLICATIONS AND MANAGEMENT

First-trimester abortion is very safe, with 0.6 deaths per 100,000 abortions, compared with childbirth that has 14 times the risk, with 8.8 deaths per 100,000 live births.[45] Overall, less than 1% of women have complications, and only 0.3% of women will have complications requiring hospitalization.[1] Complications of abortion include the following:

Hemorrhage

Hemorrhage occurs in less than 1% of terminations.[46] The definition of a postabortal hemorrhage varies among studies, making it difficult to estimate risk. The SFP considers hemorrhage as excessive bleeding requiring transfusion, hospital admission, or greater than 500 mL of blood loss. Hysterectomy for severe hemorrhage is performed in 1.4 per 10,000 abortions of any gestational age. The risk factors for hemorrhage are provider inexperience, increasing gestational age, advanced maternal age, increased parity, prior cesarean section or uterine scar, fibroids, a history of obstetric hemorrhage, and gestational age.[46] The causes include atony, abnormal placentation (extremely rare in the first trimester), cervical laceration, perforation, coagulopathy, and POC.[46] Oxytocin given routinely during a first-trimester abortion does not decrease blood loss.[47] Ultrasound use does not decrease hemorrhage.[48] See **Box 3** for a summary of treatment options.

Cervical Lacerations

The incidence of cervical laceration is approximately 2 per 1000 procedures.[15] Risk factors for cervical laceration in the first trimester are nulliparity, surgical inexperience

Box 3
Postabortal hemorrhage assessment and treatment

- Evaluate the cause of the hemorrhage and treat the cause.
  - Perform a speculum examination to assess the cervix for lacerations.
  - Ultrasound can evaluate for retained POC, blood, or free fluid concerning for perforation.
- Place a large-bore IV if one is not already in place and consider IV fluid boluses.
- Perform a bimanual uterine massage and give uterotonics.
  - Methylergonovine maleate 0.2 mg IM has a rapid onset of 5 minutes. It is contraindicated in hypertension.
  - Misoprostol 400 mcg to 800 mcg can be given sublingually, buccally, or per rectum. Sublingual (SL) misoprostol has the fastest onset, but may cause the most side effects.[43] A 400-mcg SL dose may decrease side effects. Vaginal and rectal administration of misoprostol has a somewhat slower onset than SL and a longer-lasting effect with both acting for approximately 4 hours.[43] The common side effects are shivering, nausea, pyrexia, and chills. A misoprostol fever should resolve after 3 hours.[56]
- For continued bleeding with concern for disseminated intravascular coagulation or other coagulopathy, consider evaluation by placing 10 mL of blood in a glass tube and observe for clot formation over 5 to 10 minutes.
- For severe hemorrhage, transfer to a hospital where uterine artery embolization, balloon compression techniques, laparoscopy, laparotomy, or hysterectomy should be performed.

Adapted from Kerns J, Steinauer J. Management of postabortion hemorrhage: release date November 2012 SFP guideline #20131. Contraception 2013;87(3):331–42.

and inadequate dilation. Small lacerations may resolve with pressure or silver nitrate application. Larger lacerations can be treated with Monsel solution or by suturing if they continue bleeding. If there is excessive bleeding or bleeding that continues despite repair, one should be concerned for a high laceration with possible uterine artery involvement. High lacerations may require repair by laparotomy or laparoscopy.

Uterine Perforation

Uterine perforation occurs in approximately 0.1 to 3.0 in 1000 procedures.[15] Perforations generally occur at the fundus and are more likely to cause complications if they occur after the first trimester.[4] The perforating instrument is most likely the suction cannula, followed by a dilator and then a curette.[49,50] The risk factors include provider inexperience, inadequate dilation, the use of a sound before the procedure, and increasing gestational age.[51] Instruments passing further than expected with little resistance or loss of a gritty sensation can be an indication of perforation. Women may have a sudden onset of abdominal pain associated with perforation. Bowel or omentum may be noted in the cannula. If a perforation is suspected and there is minimal blood loss and no concern for bowel involvement, patients can be monitored for 2 to 4 hours in the clinic. If patients remain stable with normal vital signs, have no peritoneal signs on serial examinations, and do not have increasing pain, then they can be discharged home with precautions for worsening symptoms. Many small perforations are likely unrecognized or clinically insignificant, with one study reporting 7 times as many perforations diagnosed with concurrent laparoscopy during the procedure than diagnosed clinically.[52] Patients with perforations with hemorrhage, concern for bowel involvement, or injury to other surrounding structures should be transferred to the hospital for laparoscopy or laparotomy.

Incomplete Abortion

Women typically present with lower abdominal pain and bleeding and possibly fever. Reaspiration for retained POC is uncommon with a first-trimester abortion. It occurs in 0.29% to 1.96% of abortions.[4] Women with heavy bleeding or infection should be reaspirated. Using ultrasound for diagnosis of retained POC can be challenging because the ultrasound findings of asymptomatic and symptomatic women can be quite similar after abortion.[53] The endometrial cavity of both groups can have similar Doppler flow, cavity irregularity, and echogenic contents, although in general the endometrial thickness of women with retained POC (15.3 mm with a range of 1.8–34.0 mm) is statistically significantly greater than those without retained POC (10.8 mm with a range of 1–29 mm).[53] Another study found that an endometrial thickness of 13 mm or greater could be used to suggest retained POC in symptomatic women.[54] Medical management with misoprostol can be considered for women who are clinically stable.[4]

Hematometra

Hematometra is an accumulation of blood in the uterus ranging from 250 to 1500 mL resulting in cramping or rectal pressure that can occur minutes to hours after a procedure.[4] Because of the large amount of blood in the uterus, women may become hypotensive or have vasovagal episodes. On clinical examination, the uterus will feel firm and large and ultrasound will reveal much blood in the uterus. Treatment is reaspiration of the uterus. Treatment with methylergonovine maleate 0.2 mg intramuscularly (IM) or misoprostol 800 mcg buccally or rectally may be given after the procedure.

Postabortal UGT Infections

UGT are uncommon, happening in less than 1% of procedures, and are decreased with preoperative doxycycline prophylaxis.[10] Infections usually occur days after the procedure and are diagnosed by fever, pain, pelvic tenderness, and leukocytosis. Women should be evaluated for possible retained POC and reaspirated if retained products are suspected. Women should be treated with antibiotics using the Centers for Disease Control and Prevention's recommendations for pelvic inflammatory disease from the "Sexually Transmitted Diseases Treatment Guidelines."[55] Women with mild disease can be treated as an outpatient.

Failed Attempted Abortion

The incidence of failed attempted abortion is 0.5 per 1000 abortions.[4] The risk is increased by early gestational age; operator inexperience; or uterine anomalies, such as fibroids, a bicornuate uterus, or a septate uterus. If unrecognized at the time of the procedure, patients usually present with ongoing pregnancy symptoms and an enlarging uterus. Women should be counseled and reaspirated or offered medication abortion if within the gestational age limits.

Vasovagal Episode

A vasovagal episode can occur during or after a procedure. Women may complain of feeling faint, dizzy, or nauseated. Treatment includes placing patients in the Trendelenburg position, placing cool compresses on their face, or smelling salts with resolution within 3 to 5 minutes. If symptoms persist despite conservative measures, patients can be given atropine 0.4 mg to 1.0 IV or IM.[4]

POSTOPERATIVE CARE

- After the procedure, warning signs should be reviewed with patients, including a temperature greater than 101°F, stronger uterine cramping, or bleeding that soaks more than 2 pads per hour for 2 hours. Misoprostol use can commonly cause fever with shivering, which will peak at 1 to 2 hours and resolve by 3 hours after use.[56]
- Women should be given a 24-hour emergency contact number in case of concerning symptoms and be advised of where to go and seek treatment if needed after hours.
- It is recommended that vaginal intercourse and tampons are avoided for 1 week after a procedure.
- Anticipatory guidance should be given to expect light bleeding for up to 2 weeks after the procedure and that patients' menses should return in 4 to 8 weeks. However, ovulation may occur before this time and postabortal contraception should be emphasized as outlined later.
- A routine follow-up visit is not needed after a procedure. Complications and continuing pregnancy were not significantly different in a study comparing routine follow-up with follow-up as needed.[57]

CONTRACEPTION

All women seeking an abortion should be offered a contraceptive method at the time of her initial evaluation. Long-acting reversible contraceptives, such as the etonogestrel implant and intrauterine device (IUD), have been found to statistically significantly decrease abortion incidence.[58] IUDs placed immediately after an abortion lower the incidence rates of repeat abortions from 34.6 per 1000 woman-years to 91.3 per 1000 woman-years in controls.[59] They are cost-effective, resulting in decreased expenditures by $111 per woman at 1 year and saved $4296 per woman at 5 years compared with interval IUD placement.[60] Immediate postabortal IUDs are safe and effective; although they have a slightly higher expulsion, ranging from 3% to 5% immediately after an abortion compared with 0% to 2.7% in interval groups, continuation at 6 months is still higher because of the poor return for interval placement.[61,62] Immediate postabortal etonogestrel implant has equivalent continuation rates as compared with interval insertion.[63] Women interested in progestin or combined hormonal contraceptives can be given a prescription before leaving the clinic to be started immediately after the procedure.[64] Oral contraceptive pill packs can also be dispensed after the procedure if they are available.

OUTCOMES

Outcomes after a first-trimester surgical abortion are excellent because of its safety and rare complications. Long-term studies do not demonstrate a risk between cervical dilation and cervical incompetence, increased risk of spontaneous abortion, or preterm delivery.[15] A study evaluating the relationship between first-trimester abortion and mental illness found that women were not more likely to have psychiatric contact after an abortion compared with before the abortion.[65] Although some states require informing women that abortion increases the risk of breast cancer, no high-quality study has found this association to be true.[66–68]

SUMMARY

Surgical abortion is a safe and common outpatient procedure with a very low incidence of complications, especially for experienced providers. Manual and electric uterine aspiration are equally effective and safe options for first-trimester surgical abortions. Preprocedure prophylaxis with doxycycline for the prevention of postabortal infection is recommended. Cervical preparation with misoprostol or osmotic dilators is not routinely recommended but should be considered at greater than 12 weeks' gestation and in select cases for adolescents or if there is difficulty with initial dilation. For first-trimester surgical abortions, ibuprofen and local anesthesia via PCB may offer sufficient pain control for many women. Women who receive IV sedation for procedures report the lowest pain scores. Immediate long-acting reversible contraceptive initiation has the potential to reduce unintended pregnancy and repeat abortion.[59] IUDs and the etonogestrel implant may be inserted immediately after the procedure. Although no routine follow-up appointment is required and complication incidence is low, women should have access to a provider after their procedure and given specific discharge information regarding when to call for signs of complications, such as infection and hemorrhage.

REFERENCES

1. Guttmacher Institute. Facts on induced abortion in the United States. 2011. Available at: http://www.guttmacher.org/pubs/fb_induced_abortion.html. Accessed April 11, 2013.
2. Jones RK, Zolna MR, Henshaw SK, et al. Abortion in the United States: incidence and access to services, 2005. Perspect Sex Reprod Health 2008; 40(1):6–16.
3. Pazol K, Creanga AA, Zane SB, et al. Abortion surveillance–United States, 2009. MMWR Surveill Summ 2012;61(8):1–44.
4. Paul M. Management of unintended and abnormal pregnancy: comprehensive abortion care. West Sussex (England): Wiley-Blackwell; 2009.
5. Moore AM, Frohwirth L, Blades N. What women want from abortion counseling in the United States: a qualitative study of abortion patients in 2008. Soc Work Health Care 2011;50(6):424–42.
6. Guiahi M, Davis A. First-trimester abortion in women with medical conditions: release date October 2012 SFP guideline #20122. Contraception 2012;86(6): 622–30.
7. Kaneshiro B, Bednarek P, Isley M, et al. Blood loss at the time of first-trimester surgical abortion in anticoagulated women. Contraception 2011; 83(5):431–5.
8. O'Connell K, Jones HE, Simon M, et al. First-trimester surgical abortion practices: a survey of National Abortion Federation members. Contraception 2009; 79(5):385–92.
9. Kulier R, Kapp N. Comprehensive analysis of the use of pre-procedure ultrasound for first- and second-trimester abortion. Contraception 2011;83(1): 30–3.
10. Achilles SL, Reeves MF, Society of Family Planning. Prevention of infection after induced abortion: release date October 2010: SFP guideline 20102. Contraception 2011;83(4):295–309.
11. Cetin A, Cetin M. Effect of deep injections of local anesthetics and basal dilatation of cervix in management of pain during legal abortions. A randomized, controlled study. Contraception 1997;56(2):85–7.
12. Heath V, Chadwick V, Cooke I, et al. Should tissue from pregnancy termination and uterine evacuation routinely be examined histologically? BJOG 2000; 107(6):727–30.

13. American Society of Anesthesiologists Task Force on S, Analgesia by N-A. Practice guidelines for sedation and analgesia by non-anesthesiologists. Anesthesiology 2002;96(4):1004–17.
14. Low N, Mueller M, Van Vliet HA, et al. Perioperative antibiotics to prevent infection after first-trimester abortion. Cochrane Database Syst Rev 2012;(3): CD005217.
15. Allen RH, Goldberg AB, Board of Society of Family Planning. Cervical dilation before first-trimester surgical abortion (<14 weeks' gestation). SFP guideline 20071. Contraception 2007;76(2):139–56.
16. Kapp N, Lohr PA, Ngo TD, et al. Cervical preparation for first trimester surgical abortion. Cochrane Database Syst Rev 2010;(2):CD007207.
17. Vimala N, Mittal S, Kumar S. Sublingual misoprostol before first trimester abortion: a comparative study using two dose regimens. Indian J Med Sci 2004; 58(2):54–61.
18. Carbonell Esteve JL, Mari JM, Valero F, et al. Sublingual versus vaginal misoprostol (400 microg) for cervical priming in first-trimester abortion: a randomized trial. Contraception 2006;74(4):328–33.
19. Saxena P, Salhan S, Sarda N. Sublingual versus vaginal route of misoprostol for cervical ripening prior to surgical termination of first trimester abortions. Eur J Obstet Gynecol Reprod Biol 2006;125(1):109–13.
20. Carbonell JL, Velazco A, Rodriguez Y, et al. Oral versus vaginal misoprostol for cervical priming in first-trimester abortion: a randomized trial. Eur J Contracept Reprod Health Care 2001;6(3):134–40.
21. Bartz D, Maurer R, Allen RH, et al. Buccal misoprostol compared with synthetic osmotic cervical dilator before surgical abortion: a randomized controlled trial. Obstet Gynecol 2013;122(1):57–63.
22. MacIsaac L, Grossman D, Balistreri E, et al. A randomized controlled trial of laminaria, oral misoprostol, and vaginal misoprostol before abortion. Obstet Gynecol 1999;93(5 Pt 1):766–70.
23. Meirik O, My Huong NT, Piaggio G, et al. Complications of first-trimester abortion by vacuum aspiration after cervical preparation with and without misoprostol: a multicentre randomised trial. Lancet 2012;379(9828):1817–24.
24. Allen RH, Fitzmaurice G, Lifford KL, et al. Oral compared with intravenous sedation for first-trimester surgical abortion: a randomized controlled trial. Obstet Gynecol 2009;113(2 Pt 1):276–83.
25. Renner RM, Jensen JT, Nichols MD, et al. Pain control in first trimester surgical abortion. Cochrane Database Syst Rev 2009;(2):CD006712.
26. Renner RM, Nichols MD, Jensen JT, et al. Paracervical block for pain control in first-trimester surgical abortion: a randomized controlled trial. Obstet Gynecol 2012;119(5):1030–7.
27. Cansino C, Edelman A, Burke A, et al. Paracervical block with combined ketorolac and lidocaine in first-trimester surgical abortion: a randomized controlled trial. Obstet Gynecol 2009;114(6):1220–6.
28. Micks EA, Edelman AB, Renner RM, et al. Hydrocodone-acetaminophen for pain control in first-trimester surgical abortion: a randomized controlled trial. Obstet Gynecol 2012;120(5):1060–9.
29. Allen RH, Kumar D, Fitzmaurice G, et al. Pain management of first-trimester surgical abortion: effects of selection of local anesthesia with and without lorazepam or intravenous sedation. Contraception 2006;74(5):407–13.
30. Wiebe ER, Byczko B, Kaczorowski J, et al. Can we safely avoid fasting before abortions with low-dose procedural sedation? A retrospective cohort chart

review of anesthesia-related complications in 47,748 abortions. Contraception 2013;87(1):51–4.
31. Guerrero JM, Castano PM, Schmidt EO, et al. Music as an auxiliary analgesic during first trimester surgical abortion: a randomized controlled trial. Contraception 2012;86(2):157–62.
32. Wu J, Chaplin W, Amico J, et al. Music for surgical abortion care study: a randomized controlled pilot study. Contraception 2012;85(5):496–502.
33. Kulier R, Fekih A, Hofmeyr GJ, et al. Surgical methods for first trimester termination of pregnancy. Cochrane Database Syst Rev 2001;(4):CD002900.
34. Bird ST, Harvey SM, Beckman LJ, et al. Similarities in women's perceptions and acceptability of manual vacuum aspiration and electric vacuum aspiration for first trimester abortion. Contraception 2003;67(3):207–12.
35. Mittal S, Sehgal R, Aggarwal S, et al. Cervical priming with misoprostol before manual vacuum aspiration versus electric vacuum aspiration for first-trimester surgical abortion. Int J Gynaecol Obstet 2011;112(1):34–9.
36. Singh RH, Ghanem KG, Burke AE, et al. Predictors and perception of pain in women undergoing first trimester surgical abortion. Contraception 2008;78(2): 155–61.
37. Hemlin J, Moller B. Manual vacuum aspiration, a safe and effective alternative in early pregnancy termination. Acta Obstet Gynecol Scand 2001;80(6):563–7.
38. Edelman A, Nichols MD, Jensen J. Comparison of pain and time of procedures with two first-trimester abortion techniques performed by residents and faculty. Am J Obstet Gynecol 2001;184(7):1564–7.
39. Lichtenberg ES, Paul M. Surgical abortion prior to 7 weeks of gestation: release date March 2013 SFP guideline #20132. Contraception 2013;88(1):7–17.
40. Dean G, Cardenas L, Darney P, et al. Acceptability of manual versus electric aspiration for first trimester abortion: a randomized trial. Contraception 2003; 67(3):201–6.
41. Baldauf JJ, Dreyfus M, Ritter J, et al. Risk of cervical stenosis after large loop excision or laser conization. Obstet Gynecol 1996;88(6):933–8.
42. Pennes DR, Bowerman RA, Silver TM, et al. Failed first trimester pregnancy termination: uterine anomaly as etiologic factor. J Clin Ultrasound 1987;15(3):165–70.
43. Tang OS, Chan CC, Ng EH, et al. A prospective, randomized, placebo-controlled trial on the use of mifepristone with sublingual or vaginal misoprostol for medical abortions of less than 9 weeks gestation. Hum Reprod 2003;18(11): 2315–8.
44. Winikoff B, Dzuba IG, Chong E, et al. Extending outpatient medical abortion services through 70 days of gestational age. Obstet Gynecol 2012;120(5):1070–6.
45. Raymond EG, Grimes DA. The comparative safety of legal induced abortion and childbirth in the United States. Obstet Gynecol 2012;119(2 Pt 1):215–9.
46. Kerns J, Steinauer J. Management of postabortion hemorrhage: release date November 2012 SFP guideline #20131. Contraception 2013;87(3):331–42.
47. Nygaard IH, Valbo A, Heide HC, et al. Is oxytocin given during surgical termination of first trimester pregnancy useful? A randomized controlled trial. Acta Obstet Gynecol Scand 2011;90(2):174–8.
48. Schulz KF, Grimes DA, Christensen DD. Vasopressin reduces blood loss from second-trimester dilatation and evacuation abortion. Lancet 1985;2(8451):353–6.
49. Chen LH, Lai SF, Lee WH, et al. Uterine perforation during elective first trimester abortions: a 13-year review. Singapore Med J 1995;36(1):63–7.
50. Mittal S, Misra SL. Uterine perforation following medical termination of pregnancy by vacuum aspiration. Int J Gynaecol Obstet 1985;23(1):45–50.

51. Grimes DA, Schulz KF, Cates WJ Jr. Prevention of uterine perforation during curettage abortion. JAMA 1984;251(16):2108–11.
52. Kaali SG, Szigetvari IA, Bartfai GS. The frequency and management of uterine perforations during first-trimester abortions. Am J Obstet Gynecol 1989; 161(2):406–8.
53. McEwing RL, Anderson NG, Meates JB, et al. Sonographic appearances of the endometrium after termination of pregnancy in asymptomatic versus symptomatic women. J Ultrasound Med 2009;28(5):579–86.
54. Ustunyurt E, Kaymak O, Iskender C, et al. Role of transvaginal sonography in the diagnosis of retained products of conception. Arch Gynecol Obstet 2008; 277(2):151–4.
55. Workowski KA, Berman S, Centers for Disease Control and Prevention (CDC). Sexually transmitted diseases treatment guidelines, 2010. MMWR Recomm Rep 2010;59(RR-12):1–110.
56. Elati A, Weeks A. Risk of fever after misoprostol for the prevention of postpartum hemorrhage: a meta-analysis. Obstet Gynecol 2012;120(5):1140–8.
57. Gatter M, Roth N, Safarian C, et al. Eliminating the routine postoperative surgical abortion visit. Contraception 2012;86(4):397–401.
58. Peipert JF, Madden T, Allsworth JE, et al. Preventing unintended pregnancies by providing no-cost contraception. Obstet Gynecol 2012;120(6):1291–7.
59. Goodman S, Hendlish SK, Reeves MF, et al. Impact of immediate postabortal insertion of intrauterine contraception on repeat abortion. Contraception 2008; 78(2):143–8.
60. Salcedo J, Sorensen A, Rodriguez MI. Cost analysis of immediate postabortal IUD insertion compared to planned IUD insertion at the time of abortion follow up. Contraception 2013;87(4):404–8.
61. Bednarek PH, Creinin MD, Reeves MF, et al. Immediate versus delayed IUD insertion after uterine aspiration. N Engl J Med 2011;364(23):2208–17.
62. Fox MC, Oat-Judge J, Severson K, et al. Immediate placement of intrauterine devices after first and second trimester pregnancy termination. Contraception 2011;83(1):34–40.
63. Madden T, Eisenberg DL, Zhao Q, et al. Continuation of the etonogestrel implant in women undergoing immediate postabortion placement. Obstet Gynecol 2012;120(5):1053–9.
64. Centers for Disease Control and Prevention (CDC). U.S. Medical eligibility criteria for contraceptive use, 2010. MMWR Recomm Rep 2010;59(RR-4):1–86.
65. Munk-Olsen T, Laursen TM, Pedersen CB, et al. Induced first-trimester abortion and risk of mental disorder. N Engl J Med 2011;364(4):332–9.
66. Rowlands S. Misinformation on abortion. Eur J Contracept Reprod Health Care 2011;16(4):233–40.
67. Committee on Gynecologic Practice. ACOG Committee opinion No. 434: induced abortion and breast cancer risk. Obstet Gynecol 2009;113(6): 1417–8.
68. Turner Richardson C, Nash E. Misinformed consent: the medical accuracy of state-developed abortion counseling materials. Guttmacher Pol'y Rev 2006; 9(4):6–11.
69. World Health Organization. Safe abortion: technical and policy guidance for health systems. 2nd edition. Geneva: WHO; 2012. Avaiable at: http://www.who.int/reproductivehealth/publications/unsafe_abortion/9789241548434/en/.
70. Royal College of Obstetricians and Gynaecologists (RCOG). The care of women requesting induced abortion. London (England): Royal College of Obstetricians

and Gynaecologists (RCOG); 2011. p. 130. Available at: http://www.rcog.org.uk/files/rcog-corp/Abortion%20guideline_web_1.pdf.
71. National Abortion Federation. 2013 Clinical policy guidelines. Washington (DC): National Abortion Federation; 2013. Available at: http://www.prochoice.org/pubs_research/publications/documents/2013NAFCPGsforweb.pdf.
72. Allen RH, Goldberg AB. Board of Society of Family Practice. Cervical dilation before first-trimester surgical abortion (<14 weeks' gestation). SFP guideline 20071. Contraception 2007;76(2):139–56.

Hysteroscopic Sterilization in the Office Setting

Kelly R. Hodges, MD[a,*], Laurie S. Swaim, MD[b]

KEYWORDS

• Sterilization • Hysteroscopy • Essure • Mircoinsert • Office • Contraception

KEY POINTS

- Essure hysteroscopic sterilization is an effective sterilization procedure that can be performed safely in the office setting.
- Keys to success in the office setting are staff preparation, appropriate patient selection, comprehensive patient counseling, completion of a preprocedure checklist, equipment availability, and patient comfort.
- Procedure success requires adherence to recommended instructions for placement of the microinserts, appropriate patient follow-up, and confirmation of bilateral tubal occlusion.

INTRODUCTION

Although multiple methods of contraception are available, surgical sterilization is one of the most popular. In the United States, female sterilization is second only to oral contraceptive pill use for the prevention of pregnancy.[1] For women who no longer desire fertility, sterilization is a safe and highly effective option.[2]

Traditional methods of female permanent sterilization (eg, laparoscopic and abdominal tubal ligation) require general or regional anesthesia, expose the patient to the intrinsic risks of a surgical procedure, and require a period of postoperative recovery. In addition, both procedures require abdominal wall incisions and, in the case of laparoscopy, introduction of trocars. Alternatively, hysteroscopic sterilization may be performed in an ambulatory setting, does not require abdominal incisions, and is associated with decreased postprocedural pain.[3]

Two methods of hysteroscopic tubal sterilization are currently approved by the U.S. Food and Drug Administration (FDA). The Essure microinsert system (Conceptus Inc, San Carlos, CA, USA) was approved in 2002, followed by the Adiana Complete Transcervical Sterilization System (Hologic, Bedford, MA, USA) in 2009. Both methods

[a] Division of Gynecologic and Obstetric Specialists, Department of Obstetrics and Gynecology, Baylor College of Medicine, 6651 Main Street, Set 1020 Houston, TX 77030, USA; [b] Division of Gynecologic and Obstetric Specialists, Baylor College of Medicine, Texas Children's Hospital, 6651 Main Street, Set 1020 Houston, TX 77030, USA

* Corresponding author.

E-mail address: krhodges@bcm.edu

Obstet Gynecol Clin N Am 40 (2013) 671–685

http://dx.doi.org/10.1016/j.ogc.2013.08.007 obgyn.theclinics.com

0889-8545/13/$ – see front matter

occlude the fallopian tubes through stimulating tissue fibrosis and subsequent scarring. Essure microinsert is currently the only method available in the United States, because Adiana is no longer manufactured.

Hysteroscopic sterilization is growing in popularity. Nearly 500,000 women have been sterilized using this method,[4] and an increasing number of physicians are now performing this procedure in the office setting.

The office setting can provide a cost-effective, convenient, and safe environment for hysteroscopic sterilization.[5,6] Patients may benefit from avoiding hospital preoperative visits, excessive laboratory evaluation, operating room wait times, and expense associated with hospital care. Physicians may improve productivity through remaining in their office or avoiding operating room delays. This article reviews office-hysteroscopic sterilization with the microinsert system (Essure).

MICROINSERT MECHANISM OF ACTION

The Essure microinsert is 4 cm long and, once deployed, expands to 1.5 to 2.0 mm in diameter to anchor into the fallopian tube wall. The insert has a stainless steel inner coil and a Nitinol (nickel-titanium) expanding outer coil that anchors the implant in the proper location. Wound in and around the inner coil are polyethylene terephthalate (PET) fibers. These PET fibers stimulate benign tissue growth that surrounds and infiltrates the device over time, resulting in the fallopian tube occlusion and permanent sterilization.

PREOPERATIVE EVALUATION AND PREPARATION

Patient Selection

Patient selection for office hysteroscopic sterilization is critical to procedure success. The most common reasons for failure are pain, poor visualization of the tubal ostia, and cervical stenosis.[10] To ensure successful sterilization with correct microinsert placement, the patient must be willing to use an alternate form of contraception for 3 months until tubal occlusion is confirmed. Patient exclusion criteria for the Essure procedure are listed in **Box 1**.

Counseling and Written Informed Consent

Women considering tubal sterilization with microinserts should be advised of the following;

- The permanent and irreversible nature of the procedure
- Alternate approaches to sterilization
- Options for long-acting reversible contraception
- The risk of placement failure
- The need for reliable birth control until confirmatory testing can be completed
- A theoretical increased risk of ectopic pregnancy before confirmation of tubal occlusion
- Possible adverse outcomes, including uterine and tubal perforation (see **Table 1**)

Before the procedure, a back-up plan should be created in the event both microinserts cannot be successfully placed. Consent for possible transfer to a facility that can support laparoscopy or laparotomy should be obtained before the procedure.

Preoperative Examination

A history and physical, including pelvic examination, should be performed. The pelvic examination is focused on size, position, and mobility of the uterus and impression of cervical patency.

Box 1
Exclusion criteria for the Essure procedure

In general

- Patient unwilling to use a reliable method of pregnancy prevention for 3 months after the procedure
- Patient unwilling or unable to undergo hysterosalpingogram (eg, severe contrast allergy)
- Patient uncertain about desire to end fertility
- Patient less than 6 weeks postpartum or post–pregnancy termination
- Presence of active or recent pelvic infection
- Known uterine anomaly or anatomic variant that may preclude adequate visualization of the tubal ostia
- Patient is immune-compromised or currently receiving chemotherapy

In the office setting

- Patients who cannot tolerate basic gynecologic procedures (eg, Papanicolaou smear)
- Patients with high levels of anxiety
- Patients with known cervical stenosis
- Patients with significant medical comorbidities that would preclude safe office surgery

Preoperative Laboratory Tests

Before surgery, a negative pregnancy test within 24 hours of the procedure is recommended.[9] No other routine testing is required.

Timing of Procedure

The success of the procedure requires adequate visualization of the tubal ostia. Patients on hormonal contraception can undergo the procedure at any time. If not using hormonal contraception, placement should occur during the follicular phase of the menstrual cycle.[11] This timing allows optimal visualization of the uterine cavity while decreasing the possibility of an early pregnancy. Microinsert placement is not recommended during the menstrual cycle. For patients not using hormonal contraception, a short course of progestin therapy may help improve visualization.

Premedication

Pretreatment with nonsteroidal anti-inflammatory drug (NSAIDs) is recommended to reduce tubal spasm, although no direct evidence proves its efficacy.[12,13] A variety of approaches have been used to help control operative pain and improve procedure success, although the preferred method is unclear. Many practitioners use Ketorolac tromethamine (30–60 mg) either intravenously or intramuscularly as the preferred NSAID. A combination of preoperative oral anxiolytics (eg, alprazolam, diazepam) and low-dose oral narcotic medication (eg, hydrocodone, meperidine) may improve patient comfort and reduce anxiety. In a large series, Arjona and colleagues[14] premedicated 1615 patients with 600 mg of ibuprofen and 10 mg of diazepam. No intravenous sedation or paracervical block was used. These investigators reported 99% bilateral placement and only 3.1% reported pain greater than a menstrual cycle. Hydroxyzine can be used to help prevent nausea and is mildly sedating. Intravenous sedation is an option in the office, but requires additional training and equipment, and increases the risk of potential complications and side effects from the medication.

Prophylactic Antibiotics

Antibiotics are not routinely administered during hysteroscopic sterilization.

CONSIDERATIONS FOR THE OFFICE PROCEDURE

Scheduling

When a physician is initiating a new office procedure, scheduling should ensure maximum office productivity. Physicians can expect the procedure to take 30 minutes and can anticipate approximately 1 hour total time for the complete patient visit. A common strategy is to perform the procedure before clinic hours or during lunch breaks, which allows normal morning and afternoon clinic flow. Another is to schedule back-to-back office procedures. Ease of scheduling, staffing, and patient flow may be facilitated when the provider performs ambulatory surgery on a predetermined day. This type of scheduling may be more appealing to anesthesia providers who may travel from office to office. Surgeons may also schedule quick office visits between cases during "turnover."

Equipment

Daily caseload limitations include equipment availability and the ability to sterilize equipment in a timely fashion. Care should be taken to sterilize equipment to promote longevity. Depending on the type of hysteroscope, gas autoclaving is preferred to steam, because the steam may damage the hysteroscope. If possible, the availability of redundant equipment ensures procedure completion in the case of malfunction or inadvertent contamination. For convenience, businesses dedicated to ambulatory surgery exist and are designed to provide anesthesia and all necessary equipment.

OFFICE PREPARATION

Practice Workflow

To facilitate an efficient, safe, and successful procedure, the office should create structured preprocedure (time-out) and procedure checklists. Samples of each are shown in **Figs. 1** and **2**.

The authors recommend the following be accomplished before the procedure day:

- Insurance preapproval and patient notification of out-of-pocket expense
- Standardized history and physical examination, laboratory tests, and imaging completed and results documented in the chart
- Procedure consent signed and placed in the chart
- The equipment checklist reviewed and necessary equipment available
- Procedure day expectations communicated with the patient, such as:
  - A ride home will be needed (preferably from a friend or family member)
  - No children should accompany the patient on procedure day
  - Comfortable clothing is recommended

Postprocedure recommendations:

- Standardized postoperative vitals sheet and operative note paperwork completed
- Instructions that include postprocedure expectations and common side effects associated with the procedure provided to the patient
- Strict sterilization and equipment handling procedures performed
- Postoperative follow-up communication shortly after the procedure

Patient Name:____

Patient Birthdate: / / MR#:______

Date of Procedure: / /

Diagnosis:____

Date of Pre-op: / /

Patient given written or website pre-op instructions: Y N Patient home escort: Y N

Name of escort:____

On Chart Prior to Surgery:

- History and Physical
- Change in medical condition since last visit: Y N
  - If so describe:____
- Signed Consent for procedure Y N
- Radiology results: Y N NA
- Pathology results: Y N NA
- Lab: UPT: + -
- Other lab:____
- Patients med list reviewed: Y N
- List all meds taken during the last 24 hours:____
- Patient allergy review

MR#__________________

Fig. 1. Preprocedure checklist.

Equipment Checklist

An equipment checklist is suggested to ensure patient safety and proper equipment availability (**Box 2**). Required elements include a 5-mm rigid hysteroscope with inflow and outflow channels and a pressure infuser for uterine distension.

Office Staff

Assisting staff members must have appropriate training in the procedure and emergency response training. If possible, 2 trained medical personnel (eg, registered nurse, or medical assistant) are recommended. One staff member may monitor the patient's vital signs and comfort, while the other is able to assist the physician with equipment and supplies as needed. However, many physicians perform this procedure with one assistant.

State Regulations

Practitioners should be aware that regulations for office procedures and office-based anesthesia vary by state, and should be reviewed before initiating office-based surgery.

Distention Medium

Normal saline is typically recommended for uterine distention during Essure placement. The isotonic solution is nontoxic, nonmetabolized, and excreted by the kidneys.

- Patient Identified with 2 identifiers
- Anesthesia assessment
- All OR medications labeled
- Equipment maintenance check
- Implants devices: type:__________________ #________________ exp:________
- Procedure Start Time: Procedure end time:
- Time out: date: time: personnel:
- Medications and dosages used: see anesthesia record
- Fluid balance (hysteroscopy): + - cc

Post Procedure:

- MA/LVN/RN assessment:
  - Post anesthesia check: anesthesia record on chart
  - Bleeding assessment: none light moderate heavy
    - If moderate or heavy MD notified:
      - Time:
      - Physician: action:
- Patient given printed or website instructions: Y N
- Instructions reviewed with patient Y N
- Follow up appointment scheduled Y N
- Follow up call 24-48 hours post op assigned Y N

Signature____________________________________Date:________________

Follow up Call: date: / / time: : comments:
Initials:

Patient Name:___________________

Fig. 2. Procedure checklist.

Box 2
General equipment checklist

- Sterile towels, drapes, and gloves
- Under-buttocks drape (with fluid pouch)
- Sterile open-sided speculum
- Sterile tenaculum or ring forceps
- Paracervical block: 27-gauge needle, 18-gauge needle, needle extender, anesthetic of choice
- Hysterosalpingogram catheter (if planning intrauterine anesthesia)
- 5-mm rigid hysteroscope with operating channel
- Camera
- 3-L saline bag and pressure bag
- Suction tubing
- Sterile dilators/os finder
- Grasper (for removal of device if incorrectly placed)

An important potential side effect of hysteroscopy is fluid overload, which may occur when liquid is instilled into the uterine cavity at a pressure that exceeds venous pressure. Fluid overload can develop rapidly, and therefore the fluid deficit should be monitored closely throughout the procedure. When the fluid deficit approaches 750 mL, the surgeon should complete the procedure expeditiously. The procedure should be terminated when the calculated fluid deficit reaches 2500 mL 0.9% normal saline.[15] If a nonionic medium is used, such as glycine, the fluid deficit should not exceed 1000 mL.

Patient Preparation

For the safety of patients and providers, maintenance of universal precautions must be followed during all surgical procedures. Although debate exists over whether hysteroscopic sterilization should be considered a sterile or clean procedure, the hysteroscope should be sterile. Povidone iodine solution is commonly used for sterile vaginal preparation. However, if the surgeon chooses to regard hysteroscopic sterilization as a clean procedure, the vulva and vagina do not need to be scrubbed.

Patient Positioning

The patient is positioned in dorsal lithotomy. Stirrups that support the legs are most comfortable, but foot stirrups will suffice if the patient is not sedated. An under-buttocks drape with fluid pouch can help monitor fluid deficit.

Anesthesia

A major obstacle to the success of office hysteroscopic sterilization is pain management. Despite the anesthetic limitations that exist for most gynecology procedures, the phase II and III prospective studies submitted for FDA approval,[12,13] and numerous subsequent studies,[3,5,16,17] have shown the Essure procedure is well tolerated by most patients when using local anesthesia with or without intravenous sedation. A recent Cochrane review noted that women reported lower pain scales during placement of the tenaculum and passage of the hysteroscope through the external and internal os when 1% lidocaine paracervical block was performed.[18] However, in the same study, women reported no decrease in pain with coil placement and paracervical block. Placement success was unaffected by the use of a paracervical block.[19]

Intrauterine local anesthetic installation has been attempted to improve analgesia at the cornua and reduce pain of coil placement. A recent review of 23 studies evaluating intrauterine anesthesia in gynecologic procedures found reduced pain in several procedures, including endometrial biopsy, curettage, and hysteroscopy.[19] However, no clear reduction in pain has been noted in studies of intrauterine anesthesia and hysteroscopic tubal occlusion.[18,19]

A vaginoscopic approach has been advocated to minimize the pain of transcervical hysteroscope insertion. With this method, the cervix is palpated and the hysteroscope manually guided into the endocervix without the use of a tenaculum or dilation. In a prospective trial, Sagiv and colleagues[20] compared the vaginoscopic approach with the "traditional" method of using a speculum, tenaculum, and anesthetic during diagnostic hysteroscopy. A visual analog scale was used to measure the intensity of pain during hysteroscopy. The mean pain score was higher in the traditional group. However, no difference was seen in patient satisfaction. Further studies are needed to evaluate the success of this method or associated pain reduction during hysteroscopic sterilization.

PROCEDURE

The procedure should begin with verification of equipment availability and cleanliness (see **Box 2**). A standard time-out should be performed using the procedure checklist. The microinsert packaging should not be opened until both ostia have been visualized and seem to be patent.

The preferred nonsteroidal anti-inflammatory drug should be administered 30 to 60 minutes before the procedure. Other oral medications, such as an anxiolytic or a narcotic, can be administered at the same time. The clinician should consider offering the patient headphones or recommend she bring her own, and these should be put on before she is positioned. A warm blanket may be placed over the patient's arms and chest for comfort.

To visualize the cervix, the authors recommend a side-opening speculum that can be removed after the hysteroscope is placed if necessary. If desired, the vagina and cervix should be prepared with iodine, and a paracervical block administered. Placement of the block prior to setting up the hysteroscopic equipment allows time for the block to set. At least 10 minutes between placement and starting the procedure is recommended.

The hysteroscope is best introduced using hydrodilation of the cervix. If hydrodilation is unsuccessful, a minimal amount of dilation is recommended to avoid fluid leakage around the hysteroscope from an overdilated cervical os. Excess force is not needed to pass the hysteroscope.

Once the uterine cavity is adequately visualized, distension must be maintained to facilitate identification of the fallopian tube ostia. Both ostia should be identified before proceeding. The introducer (found in the product packaging) is inserted into the working channel of the hysteroscope, and the hysteroscope aligned with the tubal ostia. If possible, the assistant can thread the first device delivery system into the introducer. Once threaded, the device handle and camera are held in one hand as the other continues to thread the microinsert.

For successful placement of the coils, the deployment maneuvers must be performed precisely.[11] With gentle forward movement, the microinsert delivery system is advanced into the fallopian tube until the black positioning marker on the delivery catheter reaches the fallopian tube ostium (**Fig. 3**).

Before the device is deployed, the handle of the microinsert must be stabilized against the hysteroscope or camera to prevent movement. The thumbwheel is then be rotated in the direction of the surgeon until the wheel no longer rotates (this causes

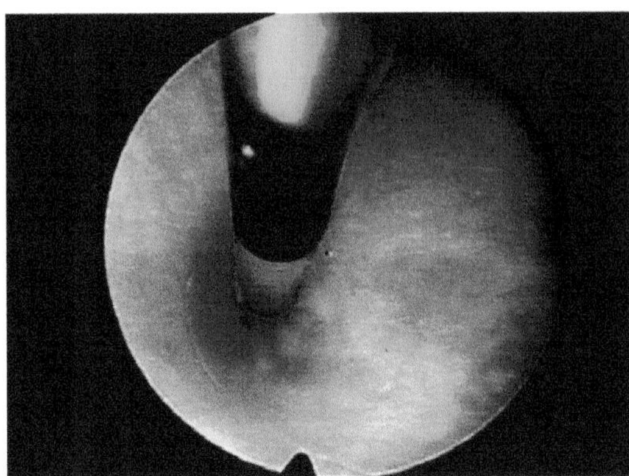

Fig. 3. Black positioning marker on the microinsert delivery catheter.

retraction of the delivery catheter, exposing the microinsert). The black positioning marker will move away from the tubal ostium toward the surgeon and disappear into the operating channel. The gold marker band should be aligned just outside the ostium. The surgeon may need to gently retract the delivery system for proper alignment (**Fig. 4**). The button on the delivery handle is pressed, and then the thumbwheel rotated toward the surgeon until no further rotation is possible (the expanded coils should be visible).

The delivery system is then removed from the operating channel and the position of the microinsert assessed; 3 to 8 expanded outer coils should be visible in the uterus.

The procedure should be repeated on the contralateral tube. Each ostia should be photographed and the number of coils present should be documented in the procedure note (**Fig. 5**).

COMPLICATIONS AND MANAGEMENT

Adverse Events

Clinical trials have shown that the most common immediate adverse reaction to the placement of Essure is abdominal cramping. Other adverse events on the day of placement and within the first year are listed in **Table 1**.[7,8]

In the same trials, tubal perforation (1%–3%), intraperitoneal placement (0.5%–3%), other unsatisfactory placement (0.5%), and coil expulsion (0.4%–2.2%) prevented reliance on Essure for sterilization. In a recent retrospective study of 4306 women who underwent Essure, 19 women experienced expulsion of one microinsert. Most expulsions were detected before or during the 3-month follow-up period.[7]

Nickel Hypersensitivity

The Essure microinsert is composed of a nickel-containing coil. Nickel hypersensitivity was considered a contraindication to the procedure when the device was first approved. However, the reported incidence of adverse events related to nickel hypersensitivity is very low (0.01%).[8] Thus, in 2011 this contraindication was removed from the Essure Instructions for Use. However, patients should still be counseled that the device does contain small amounts of nickel, which are likely not clinically significant.[9]

Trouble-Shooting Coil Placement

The Essure instructions for use do not recommend microinsert removal hysteroscopically once the insert is deployed. However, if 18 or greater coils are noted in the uterine

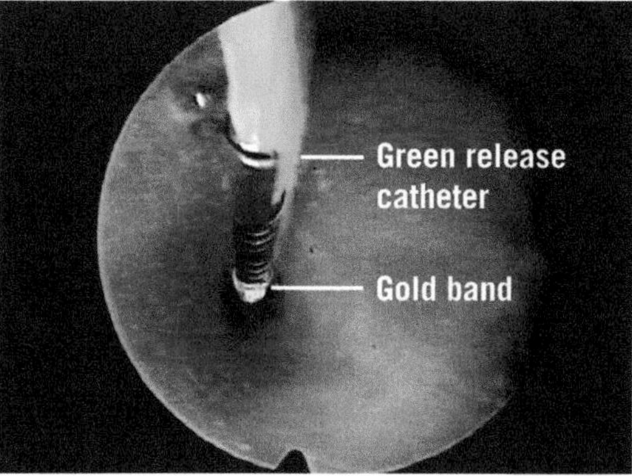

Fig. 4. Gold band alignment with tubal ostium.

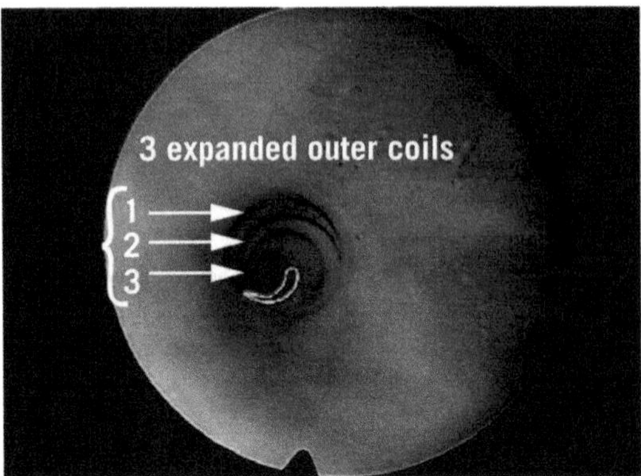

Fig. 5. Outer coils at the tubal ostia post placement.

cavity or the entire insert is deployed into the uterine cavity, hysteroscopic coil removal may be attempted at the time of insertion.[9]

Nonvisualization of coils at the tubal ostia may be the result of deep placement or deployment failure. Therefore, if no coils are visible in the tubal ostia after deployment, the delivery system should be removed and examined for the presence of coils (**Fig. 6**).

Management of Unsuccessful Microinsert Placement

Reported rates of successful placement of microinserts range from 88% to 98%.[7,12,13,21] However, several factors, such as proximal tubal occlusion, tubal stenosis, tortuosity, or tubal spasm, can make placement impossible despite proper technique. In addition, these same factors increase the risk of tubal or uterine perforation.

Failed placement

When failed placement occurs because of difficulties visualizing or accessing the tubal lumen, or because of presumed tubal spasm, a repeat attempt at a future date is reasonable. In one trial, bilateral placement was accomplished with one procedure in 446 of 507 women, and an additional 18 women during a second procedure.[12]

Perforation or migration

Perforation and migration of the microinsert are uncommon complications. In several case studies of uterine or tubal perforation or coil migration,[22–24] the complication was easily managed with laparoscopic removal of the coil. However, removal of the perforated coil may be challenging, because the device may be associated with significant adhesions or fixation onto local structures.[25–27]

Table 1
Adverse events

Day of Placement	First Year
Abdominal cramping (30%)	Back pain (9%)
Pain (1%–13%)	Dyspareunia (4%)
Nausea or vomiting (11%)	Dysmenorrhea (3%)
Dizziness or feeling light headed (9%)	Pelvic pain (2.5%)
Bleeding or spotting (7%)	–

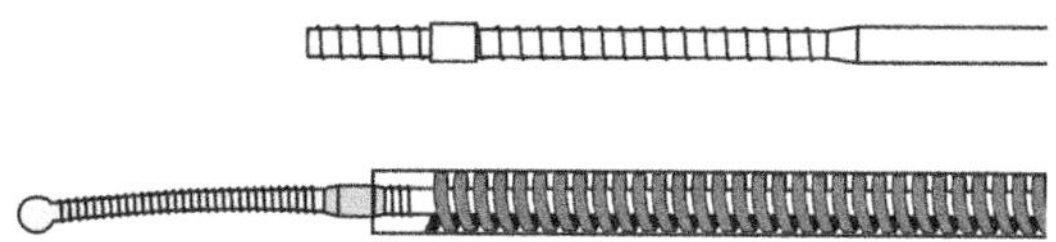

Fig. 6. Delivery system with and without microinsert.

In addition, the microinsert may conduct energy and cause injury to surrounding tissues if contacted by an electrosurgical source. Therefore, electrosurgery at the uterine cornua and proximal fallopian tubes must be approached with caution.[9]

In a prospective study of 33 microinsert procedures, Valle and colleagues,[28] reported that coil perforation occurred during procedures described as uncomplicated. However, Thoma and colleagues[22] described 2 signs noted during a placement with confirmed perforation. First, during the release, the black positioning marker on the delivery catheter did not retract toward the surgeon. The investigators theorized that this may occur when the coil is not free in the tubal lumen, but anchored because of perforation. Second, at the moment of detachment of the delivery wire from the coil, the coil seemed to be "sucked in by the tube," which may represent excess expansion of the coil in the abdominal cavity. Microinsert placement should never require force. The procedure should be terminated if gentle traction fails to advance the device.

Immediate laparoscopic inspection for symptom-free patients with suspected perforation is not recommended. The patient should be made aware of the events during the procedure and counseled to report significant abdominal pain or fever. In addition, adequate birth control and follow-up hysterosalpingogram are imperative.

Fluid Management

Given the brevity of the Essure procedure, fluid overload should be a rare complication. In rare instances, fluid overload can be associated with hyponatremia and congestive heart failure. Nausea, malaise, and headache are early symptoms of hyponatremia.[29] If fluid overload is suspected, transfer to an acute care facility for monitoring, correction of electrolyte imbalance, and diuresis is imperative.

Patient Discomfort

Patient comfort and cooperation are of utmost importance to the safety and completion of the procedure. The procedure should be terminated if the patient cannot tolerate the surgery.

Vasovagal Syncope

Manipulation and dilation of the cervix is associated with vasovagal syncope. A retrospective review of 4306 women during outpatient Essure procedures showed an incidence of vasovagal side effects in 2% of patients.[7] Preceding syncope, a patient may complain of tunnel vision, dizziness, nausea, pallor, or diaphoresis. Rapid intervention is facilitated by staff familiar with these signs and symptoms. Use of the Trendelenburg position, if possible, is almost always curative. Recovery after a vasovagal episode begins soon after fainting and generally occurs in less than a minute. In rare cases, atropine (0.5 mg) can be used to improve symptoms. If a syncopal event occurs, the patient should remain supine for 15 to 30 minutes, because syncope can recur if the patient stands too soon after the event. The patient should have nothing by mouth until fully recovered.

POSTOPERATIVE CARE

The authors recommend the monitoring of the patient in the office for bleeding and pain for 30–60 minutes postoperatively. Clinicians should ensure that an adult is available to take the patient home after the procedure. Before discharging the patient, the clinician must review the side effects and common postoperative symptoms, including cramping, pain, nausea, vomiting, dizziness, vaginal bleeding, or vaginal spotting. The patient should not have vomiting or frank vaginal bleeding. Return to normal activity is anticipated in one day or less for most patients.

The authors recommend monitoring postprocedure pain and bleeding; this can be easily accomplished with a follow-up phone call the day of the procedure and 1 or 2 days postprocedure. Patients appreciate the follow-up, and physicians have the opportunity to assess the pain control techniques. Abnormal or worrisome findings may be managed early. Patients should be instructed to continue birth control for 3 months until confirmatory hysterosalpingogram can be performed.

Postprocedure Confirmation

The FDA recommends hysterosalpingogram for the confirmation of bilateral tubal occlusion after the Essure procedure. However, hysterosalpingogram is painful, time-consuming, and expensive, which may account for poor compliance. Studies have shown hysterosalpingogram rates as low as 12.5% in counseled women receiving care at a University clinic.[25] The hysterosalpingogram should be performed at least 3 months after the Essure procedure, because scarring and occlusion are expected to be complete by this time.

Several studies recently showed the importance of the evaluation of tubal patency. A review of hysterosalpingograms performed in 235 women after Essure placement found more than 6% revealed nonocclusion, half of which were deemed to be in the appropriate location radiographically.[26] A recent retrospective cohort study of 203 women after successful hysteroscopic placement of Essure microinserts showed complete occlusion in only 83.9% at 90 days. Those women with tubal patency at initial hysterosalpingogram had a repeat hysterosalpingogram 6 months after insert placement, which revealed occlusion rates of 94.2%.[27] Difficult placement of the microinserts has been associated with improper position on follow-up imaging.[30]

Ultrasound has been proposed as a method to determine correct implant placement after hysteroscopic sterilization. Charts of more than 600 women were retrospectively reviewed after Essure placement and 3-dimensional ultrasound follow-up. The location and shape of the inserts was determined to be normal in 86%.[31] European researchers have suggested that the use of 3-dimensional ultrasound for the assessment of inserts can decrease the number of hysterosalpingograms required to determine placement. In their retrospective review, Legendre and colleagues[32] compared the need for hysterosalpingogram after 2-dimensional and 3-dimensional ultrasound in women who underwent the Essure procedure. Most inserts (>99%) were visualized by 3-dimensional ultrasound, and hysterosalpingogram was only required in 14% in whom the insert was in the distal tube, compared with 27% in those screened with 2-dimensional ultrasound.

HSG is the current gold standard for demonstration of tubal occlusion. Ultrasound may be an option to confirm tubal occlusion but further studies are needed to assess its effectiveness.

OUTCOMES

Patient satisfaction is high after hysteroscopic sterilization in terms of placement of the device and contraceptive efficacy.[14,17,33] Successful bilateral placement of Essure microinserts is reported at approximately 88% to 98%.[7,12,13,21] A retrospective review of more than 800 hysteroscopic sterilization procedures found successful bilateral microinsert placement and bilateral tubal occlusion in 96.2% and 93.0% of Essure procedures, respectively. In practice, the actual non-placement rate of Essure may be as high as 10% and tubal occlusion is delayed by many months in a small percentage of women with appropriate placement. Failure to successfully occlude bilateral fallopian tubes via laparascopy is rare (<2%). Women should be counseled that compared to laparoscopic sterilization, hysteroscopic sterilization is associated with a higher initial failure rate.[34]

Efficacy

Conceptus Inc. reports that in woman who had tubal occlusion confirmed with hysterosalpingogram, the efficacy of the Essure microinsert system for preventing pregnancy at 5 years is 99.83%. Most failures occurred before hysterosalpingogram confirmation of tubal occlusion.[35]

Cost

Cost data are proprietary, because contractual agreements between suppliers and users may vary. The devices may be purchased as single systems; however, volume discounts have been available to purchasers. The Dry Flow Introducers are also available under separate packaging.

REFERENCES

1. Jones J, Mosher W, Daniels K. Current contraceptive use in the United States 2006–2010, and changes in patterns of use since 1995. Natl Health Stat Report 2012;60:2–26.
2. Smith RD. Contemporary hysteroscopic methods for female sterilization. Int J Gynaecol Obstet 2010;108(1):79–84.
3. Syed R, Levy J, Childers ME. Pain associated with hysteroscopic sterilization. JSLS 2007;11(1):63–5.
4. Newsire PR. Woman Care Global signs agreement with Conceptus, Inc. for exclusive distribution of Essure. Available at: http://www.prnewswire.com/news-releases/womancare-global-signs-agreement-with-conceptus-inc-for-exclusive-distribution-of-essure-113208519.html. Accessed September 22, 2013.
5. Nichols M, Carter JF, Fylstra DL, et al. A comparative study of hysteroscopic sterilization performed in-office versus a hospital operating room. J Minim Invasive Gynecol 2006;13(5):447–50.
6. Litta P, Cosmi E, Sacco G, et al. Hysteroscopic permanent tubal sterilization using a nitinol-Dacron intratubal device without anaesthesia in the outpatient setting: procedure feasibility and effectiveness. Hum Reprod 2005;20(12):3419–22.
7. Povedano B, Arjona JE, Velasco E, et al. Complications of hysteroscopic Essure((R)) sterilisation: report on 4306 procedures performed in a single centre. BJOG 2012;119(7):795–9.
8. Zurawin RK, Zurawin JL. Adverse events due to suspected nickel hypersensitivity in patients with Essure micro-inserts. J Minim Invasive Gynecol 2011;18(4): 475–82.
9. Essure: instructions for use. Available at: www.fda.gov/ohrms/dockets/ac/02/briefing/3881b1_03.pdf. Accessed September 22, 2013.
10. Readman E, Maher PJ. Pain relief and outpatient hysteroscopy: a literature review. J Am Assoc Gynecol Laparosc 2004;11(3):315–9.

11. Cooper JM. Hysteroscopic sterilization. Clin Obstet Gynecol 1992;35(2):282–98.
12. Cooper JM, Carignan CS, Cher D, et al. Microinsert nonincisional hysteroscopic sterilization. Obstet Gynecol 2003;102(1):59–67.
13. Kerin JF, Cooper JM, Price T, et al. Hysteroscopic sterilization using a micro-insert device: results of a multicentre Phase II study. Hum Reprod 2003;18(6):1223–30.
14. Arjona JE, Mino M, Cordon J, et al. Satisfaction and tolerance with office hysteroscopic tubal sterilization. Fertil Steril 2008;90(4):1182–6.
15. Loffer FD, Bradley LD, Brill AI, et al. Hysteroscopic fluid monitoring guidelines. The ad hoc committee on hysteroscopic training guidelines of the American Association of Gynecologic Laparoscopists. J Am Assoc Gynecol Laparosc 2000; 7(1):167–8.
16. Sinha D, Kalathy V, Gupta JK, et al. The feasibility, success and patient satisfaction associated with outpatient hysteroscopic sterilisation. BJOG 2007;114(6): 676–83.
17. Mino M, Arjona JE, Cordon J, et al. Success rate and patient satisfaction with the Essure sterilisation in an outpatient setting: a prospective study of 857 women. BJOG 2007;114(6):763–6.
18. Kaneshiro B, Grimes DA, Lopez LM. Pain management for tubal sterilization by hysteroscopy. Cochrane Database Syst Rev 2012;(8):CD009251.
19. Mercier RJ, Zerden ML. Intrauterine anesthesia for gynecologic procedures: a systematic review. Obstet Gynecol 2012;120(3):669–77.
20. Sagiv R, Sadan O, Boaz M, et al. A new approach to office hysteroscopy compared with traditional hysteroscopy: a randomized controlled trial. Obstet Gynecol 2006;108(2):387–92.
21. Panel P, Grosdemouge I. Predictive factors of Essure implant placement failure: prospective, multicenter study of 495 patients. Fertil Steril 2010;93(1):29–34.
22. Thoma V, Chua I, Garbin O, et al. Tubal perforation by ESSURE microinsert. J Minim Invasive Gynecol 2006;13(2):161–3.
23. Hur HC, Mansuria SM, Chen BA, et al. Laparoscopic management of hysteroscopic Essure sterilization complications: report of 3 cases. J Minim Invasive Gynecol 2008;15(3):362–5.
24. Belotte J, Shavell VI, Awonuga AO, et al. Small bowel obstruction subsequent to Essure microinsert sterilization: a case report. Fertil Steril 2011;96(1):e4–6.
25. Shavell VI, Abdallah ME, Diamond MP, et al. Post-Essure hysterosalpingography compliance in a clinic population. J Minim Invasive Gynecol 2008;15(4):431–4.
26. Lazarus E, Lourenco AP, Casper S, et al. Necessity of hysterosalpingography after Essure microinsert placement for contraception. AJR Am J Roentgenol 2012; 198(6):1460–3.
27. Rodriguez AM, Kilic GS, Vu TP, et al. Analysis of tubal patency after essure placement. J Minim Invasive Gynecol 2013;20(4):468–72.
28. Valle RF, Carignan CS, Wright TC, et al. Tissue response to the STOP microcoil transcervical permanent contraceptive device: results from a prehysterectomy study. Fertil Steril 2001;76(5):974–80.
29. Rose BD, Post TW. Clinical physiology of acid-base and electrolyte disorders. 5th edition. New York: McGraw-Hill; 2001.
30. Gerritse MB, Veersema S, Timmermans A, et al. Incorrect position of Essure microinserts 3 months after successful bilateral placement. Fertil Steril 2009;91(3): 930.e1–5.
31. Thiel J, Suchet I, Tyson N, et al. Outcomes in the ultrasound follow-up of the Essure micro-insert: complications and proper placement. J Obstet Gynaecol Can 2011;33(2):134–8.

32. Legendre G, Levaillant JM, Faivre E, et al. 3D ultrasound to assess the position of tubal sterilization microinserts. Hum Reprod 2011;26(10):2683–9.
33. Scarabin C, Dhainaut C. The ESTHYME study. Women's satisfaction after hysteroscopic sterilization (Essure micro-insert). A retrospective multicenter survey. Gynecol Obstet Fertil 2007;35(11):1123–8 [in French].
34. Savage UK, Masters SJ, Smid MC, et al. Hysteroscopic sterilization in a large group practice: experience and effectiveness. Obstet Gynecol 2009;114(6): 1227–31.
35. Clinical Data. Essure Web site. Available at: http://www.essuremd.com/about-essure/clinical-data2013. Accessed April, 2013.

Global Ablation Techniques

Sarah Woods, MD[a], Betsy Taylor, MD[b,*]

KEYWORDS

• Global ablation • Techniques • Endometrial ablation • Menorrhagia

KEY POINTS

- Global endometrial ablation is a safe uterine-sparing treatment of menorrhagia in a premenopausal patient population.
- Patient selection and counseling are key elements when deciding to proceed with global endometrial ablation in an office setting.
- The risks, benefits, and postoperative expectations must be carefully reviewed with each patient.

INTRODUCTION: NATURE OF THE PROBLEM

Global endometrial ablation techniques are a relatively new surgical technology in the arsenal for the treatment of heavy menstrual bleeding that can now be used even in an outpatient clinic setting. Before the introduction of global ablation systems, endometrial ablation was performed using a hysteroscopic approach with either a resectoscope or rollerball. A comparison of global ablation versus earlier ablation technologies notes no significant differences in success rates and some improvement in patient satisfaction.[1]

The advantages of the newer global endometrial ablation systems include less operative time, improved recovery time, as well as decreased anesthetic risk. Ablation procedures performed in an outpatient surgical or clinic setting provide advantages both of potential cost savings for patients and the health care system as well as improved patient convenience.[2]

Endometrial ablation removes or destroys the functional endometrium to the level of the basalis. Various energy sources have been used to achieve this goal, and techniques are variable in terms of success rates and operative times. Five global ablation systems are currently available for use within the United States (**Table 1**). The ease of use of these systems compared with historical ablation techniques has allowed ablation to become a widely practiced treatment of menorrhagia.

[a] Department of Obstetrics and Gynecology, University of Tennessee Health Science Center, 853 Jefferson Avenue, Rm E102, Memphis, TN 38163, USA; [b] Department of Obstetrics & Gynecology, University of New Mexico Health Sciences Center, MSC 10 5580, 1 University of New Mexico, Albuquerque, NM 87131, USA
* Corresponding author.
E-mail address: btaylor@salud.unm.edu

Obstet Gynecol Clin N Am 40 (2013) 687–695
http://dx.doi.org/10.1016/j.ogc.2013.09.001
obgyn.theclinics.com

Table 1
Global ablation systems available in the United States

	ThermaChoice I, II, and III (Gynecare, Somerville, NJ)	Her Option Cryoablator (American Medical Systems, Minnetonka, MN)	Hydro Therm Ablator (Boston Scientific, San Diego, CA)	Novasure (Cytyc, Marlborough, MA)	Microsulis Endometrial Ablation, MEA (Microsulis Americas Inc, Boca Raton, FL)
Energy source	Thermal balloon	Cryoablation	Hydrothermal	Radiofrequency electrosurgical	Microwave energy
Performed under hysteroscopic visualization	No	No	Yes	No	No
Cervical dilation (mm)	5	5	8	8	8.5
Cavity limits (cm)	4–10	$\leq$10	$\leq$10.5	6–10	6–12 vs 14
Treatment time (min)	8	10–18	10	1.5	3.5
Need for pretreatment of endometrium	3-min suction curettage	GnRH agonist	GnRH agonist	None	GnRH agonist
Device specific recommendations	Do not use in presence of • Submucosal myomas • Prior endometrial ablation • Uterine cavity volume >30 mL or <2 mL	Do not use in presence of • Polyps • Intramural leiomyomata >2 cm	Do not use in presence of • Submucosal myomas • Polyps • Intramural leiomyomata >4 cm	Do not use in presence of • Submucosal myomas • Polyps >2 cm	Preoperative ultrasound to confirm uterine wall thickness $\geq$10 mm Do not use in patients with Essure (Conceptus Inc, Mountain View, CA) Do not perform mechanical D&C at the time of ablation Confirm intact uterine cavity with hysteroscopy before device insertion
FDA approval	1997	2001	2001	2001	2003

Abbreviations: D&C, dilation and curettage; FDA, Food and Drug Administration; GnRH, Gonadotropin-releasing hormone.

INDICATIONS/CONTRAINDICATIONS

Global endometrial ablation is indicated for use in premenopausal women with menorrhagia of benign cause who no longer desire fertility (**Table 2**). Usually, patients have already tried a medical treatment and experienced ongoing problems with heavy bleeding. Patients who cannot use medical management either because of intolerance of the medications or contraindications to using hormonal methods are also appropriate candidates for ablation. Patients must be willing to accept a normalized menstruation pattern rather than expecting amenorrhea.

A thorough workup for the cause of menorrhagia is required before proceeding to ablation, including endometrial biopsy to exclude endometrial hyperplasia or malignancy. The anatomy of the endometrial cavity must also be evaluated before proceeding with ablation. This evaluation is specific to each global ablation device. Once the decision has been made to proceed with ablation, the history and physical examination and, in some cases, imaging will dictate the appropriate global ablation system to use. Additionally, the patients' history, physical examination, and preference will dictate whether an office-based procedure is appropriate.

Contraindications to global endometrial ablation include endometrial hyperplasia or cancer, current pregnancy, or current use of an intrauterine device. Patients who desire future fertility are also not candidates for endometrial ablation. Patients with an acute pelvic infection should not be offered ablation while the infection is being treated. Endometrial ablation alone does not provide contraception, so a long-term contraceptive plan should be established during the preoperative assessment.

Additional precautions or relative contraindications include the presence of fibroids, a large uterine cavity size, or müllerian anomalies. Patients with significant dysmenorrhea may not have a resolution of their pain symptoms and should be counseled appropriately. According to the Food and Drug Administration (FDA), hysteroscopic tubal sterilization should not be performed concomitantly with endometrial ablation. Postmenopausal bleeding should not be treated with global endometrial ablation.

Prior uterine surgery results in a thinner uterine wall and could potentially put intra-abdominal structures (ie, bowel and bladder) at risk for intraoperative injury. Because myomectomy and classic cesarean section may result in thinning of the myometrium, a history of these procedures is considered a contraindication to global endometrial ablation. A recent retrospective cohort explored the safety of global endometrial ablation using the Novasure (Cytyc, Marlborough, MA) and ThermaChoice (Gynecare,

Table 2
Indications/Contraindications

Indications	Contraindications	Relative Contraindications/ Precautions
Menorrhagia • Premenopausal • No desire for fertility • Willing to accept normalization of menstrual flow	Pregnancy Endometrial malignancy or hyperplasia Active or recent uterine infection Intrauterine device in place	Fibroids[a] Uterine size[a] Dysmenorrhea Müllerian anomalies Prior uterine surgery Prior Essure (Conceptus Inc, Mountain View, CA)[a] Risk factors for developing endometrial cancer

[a] System specific recommendations.

Somerville, NJ) on 162 women with 1 or more cesarean sections and concluded that efficacy and safety are comparable, but they commented on the importance of hysteroscopic cavity assessment before ablation.[3] Despite this, it is important to note that serious urinary tract injuries have been reported in women with prior cesarean sections.[4,5] The absolute number of prior cesarean sections that precludes ablation has not been determined.

PERFORMING THE PROCEDURE

- Preoperative evaluation
  - Endometrial sampling
  - Uterine cavity assessment (transvaginal ultrasound, saline infusion sonography, or office hysteroscopy)
  - Perioperative risk assessment
  - Discussion of desired anesthesia
- Preoperative considerations
  - Endometrial preparation (device specific)
  - Cervical preparation may be helpful (patient specific)
  - Informed consent
- Procedure
  - No antibiotic prophylaxis recommended
  - Surgical time out
  - Anesthesia
    - Nonsteroidal antiinflammatory drugs at least 1 hour preoperatively (helpful to reduce postoperative pain)
    - Local anesthesia with or without sedation
  - Operative steps
    - Place patients in dorsal lithotomy position
    - Place the speculum, tenaculum, and cervical dilators as necessary
    - Perform the global ablation per the recommended steps specific to the device
  - Postoperative care
    - Monitor patients after the procedure as appropriate for the level of anesthesia received
    - Counsel patients that common side effects include cramping, vaginal discharge, and light bleeding

COMPLICATIONS AND MANAGEMENT

Global endometrial ablation procedures are considered safe with minimal and acceptable risks, making them attractive to both providers and patients. All of the current systems have reported intraoperative uterine perforation and nontarget tissue thermal injury.[4,6] The original FDA trials of the current global ablation systems note the overall rate of postoperative adverse events within the first 2 weeks is less than 3% when looking at infectious morbidity, thermal injury, abdominal pain, and hematometra.[7,8] Despite this low risk for postoperative infections, case reports of serious infections have been described as far as 50 days out from the procedure.[9,10] The management of postoperative infections is related to the type of infection. Currently, the American College of Obstetricians and Gynecologists recommends against using intraoperative antibiotics for transcervical procedures.[11] Per a recent Cochrane review, there is no evidence to support or discourage the use of intraoperative antibiotics for global ablation procedures.[12]

Despite the favorable safety profile, serious and fatal complications have occurred related to unrecognized mechanical or thermal injury to nontarget tissues and/or infectious causes (**Table 3**). A review of the Manufacturer and User Facility Device Experience database from 2005 to 2011 notes that bowel injury was the most commonly reported life-threatening injury, followed by sepsis. A total of 4 deaths have been reported: 2 after radiofrequency ablation related to pulmonary embolism and sepsis, 1 after thermal balloon ablation related to bowel injury, and 1 after cryoablation related to sepsis. Up to 8% of the reported serious adverse events occurred when the ablation systems were being used outside of the manufacturers' labeled instructions.[10]

Providers who perform these procedures must be aware of these potential complications as well as the ways to prevent and quickly detect them to ensure patient safety. Each device is unique in terms of the mechanism of action and built-in safety mechanisms to avoid nontarget thermal injury. It is imperative to follow the manufacturers' labeled instructions for use. Additionally, surgical counseling and informed consent should reflect the existing risks because it may be inferred that procedures that can be performed in a clinic setting are safer. A preprocedure safety checklist is advisable and should be reviewed at the time of the procedural time out.

Late Complications

Several late postoperative complications have emerged since the advent of endometrial ablation procedures and can occur with any of the current systems.[10,13,14] All of these complications relate to the potential scarring and adhesion formation within the endometrial cavity and the possible residual or regenerated endometrial tissue.

Chronic pelvic pain and dysmenorrhea following ablation are not uncommon and can be associated with hematometra, either central or cornual and/or retrograde menstruation.[14] The findings of a retrospective cohort of 67 women who underwent

Table 3
Complications

Intraoperative	Distention media fluid overload Uterine trauma Lower-tract thermal injury Bowel injury (mechanical and thermal) Device malfunction
Postoperative/early onset	Infection • Fever • Urinary tract • Vaginal • Endometritis • Bacteremia Thermal injury Bowel injury (mechanical and thermal) Abdominal pain Death
Late onset	Postablation tubal ligation syndrome Hematometra Late-onset infection Pregnancy Delayed diagnosis of endometrial cancer

Data from Refs.[8,10,30]

hysterectomy following global endometrial ablation highlight the significance of hematometra, with 26% of the specimens from the women who had hysterectomy secondary to pain notable for hematometra.[15] Women who develop cyclic pelvic pain after ablation in combination with a history of tubal ligation and hematosalpinx have postablation tubal sterilization syndrome (PATSS).[16] PATSS has an estimated incidence as high as 10%, can develop in months to years after ablation, and usually requires definitive management with hysterectomy and salpingectomy.[17]

Pregnancies have occurred following global endometrial ablation procedures; despite some successful pregnancies, these gestations should be considered high risk for complications.[13] Case reports and small case series cite an increased risk for ectopic pregnancy, miscarriage, preterm labor, preterm premature rupture of membranes, uterine rupture, abnormal placentation, cesarean section, and postpartum hemorrhage.[18,19] Specific fetal risks have also been identified in case reports, specifically intrauterine growth restriction, amniotic band syndrome, and arthrogryposis.[18] Again, emphasis must be placed on long-term contraception when patients are considering global endometrial ablation and should be part of a preprocedural checklist.

There are patients who, despite a negative endometrial biopsy before ablation, remain at a high risk for abnormal endometrial pathology. It should be mentioned that treating these high-risk women with an ablation could mask early symptoms of endometrial cancer and make endometrial sampling more difficult in the future. The incidence of cancer following ablation among women with normal preablation pathology is likely low. A recent case report and review of the English literature revealed 22 cases of endometrial cancer after endometrial ablation, with 2 of those cases occurring after the use of a global endometrial ablation system, radiofrequency ablation, and thermal balloon ablation.[20]

OUTCOMES

Patients and providers should not expect amenorrhea because this is the outcome less than 55% of the time at 12 months after the procedure.[8] Procedural success is often measured by patient satisfaction in the months to years following the procedure. The original outcomes data for global endometrial ablation procedures are from the operating room setting. Patient satisfaction is uniformly high in the 12 months after the procedure, ranging from 86% to 99 % in the original FDA trials.[8]

All current systems have been compared in randomized clinical trials with resectoscope and/or rollerball ablation, and no significant differences in relation to patient satisfaction were found.[1] This Cochrane review highlights the difficulty of comparing techniques because a variety of outcome measures were used to determine success and patient satisfaction. Additionally, the participant groups varied in perimenopausal state and the presence of uterine fibroids. The findings from a more recent meta-analysis agreed with the Cochrane review and additionally highlighted the advantages over "first generation techniques in terms of lower operative complications, shorter operative times, and anesthetic choice."[21]

Trials comparing various global ablation systems in the outpatient setting are lacking. One randomized trial comparing radiofrequency ablation with thermal balloon ablation noted similar rates of amenorrhea at 6 months after the procedure, 39% versus 21% ($P = .1$), and similar improvement in quality-of-life measures; but radiofrequency ablation did have a shorter operative time (6.2 minutes less, $P<.001$). Greater than 90% of the patients reported improvement in their symptom of heavy bleeding at

12 months after the procedure, with only 5% undergoing further surgical intervention within the first year after ablation.[22]

Endometrial ablation has also been compared with the levonorgestrel-intrauterine system, and there is no difference in patient satisfaction at 1 and 2 years.[23] A cost-effectiveness study comparing the thermal balloon ablation and levonorgestrel-intrauterine system concluded that given the similar quality-of-life improvements, the levonorgestrel-intrauterine system is more cost-effective.[24]

Despite high patient satisfaction, there is evidence of a high reoperation rate in the 4 to 5 years after global ablation, as high as 38%.[25,26] When compared with hysterectomy, improvement in bleeding and patient satisfaction are less; despite an initial significant cost savings with ablation procedures, the cost difference narrows over time given the high need for retreatment.[7,27] Definitive surgical management with hysterectomy does carry higher rates of complications, longer operating time, and recovery time.

Patient selection is an important aspect when predicting success rates. Factors known to affect procedural success include being older than 45 years, parity of 5 or more, history of dysmenorrhea, prior tubal sterilization, and imaging suggestive of adenomyosis.[28,29] Treatment failure is an indication to proceed with definitive surgical management. Repeat ablation by the current systems is not FDA approved and would be considered an off-label use.

CURRENT CONTROVERSIES/FUTURE CONSIDERATIONS

Anesthetic choice for women undergoing global endometrial ablation in a clinic setting does need further exploration to determine an adequate pain-management strategy. The recent trial comparing bipolar radiofrequency with thermal balloon endometrial ablation in the office noted that 2 procedures in the thermal balloon group were aborted intraoperatively secondary to patient discomfort. Additionally, they reported that greater than one-third of women would have preferred general anesthesia in hindsight.[22]

It deserves mention that practitioners who desire to provide office global ablation to their patients need to have a clinic practice that can support its safe performance. All clinic staff will need to be involved with training and the appropriate maintenance of certification to be prepared for any, although likely rare, adverse outcomes or complications that could arise from the anesthesia administration and/or the procedure itself.

SUMMARY

Global endometrial ablation is a safe uterine-sparing treatment of menorrhagia in a premenopausal patient population. Patient selection and counseling are key elements when deciding to proceed with a global endometrial ablation in an office setting. The risks, benefits, and postoperative expectations must be carefully reviewed with each patient.

REFERENCES

1. Lethaby A, Hickey M, Garry R, et al. Endometrial resection/ablation techniques for heavy menstrual bleeding. Cochrane Database Syst Rev 2009;(4):CD001501.
2. Marsh F, Kremer C, Duffy S. Delivering an effective outpatient service in gynaecology. A randomised controlled trial analysing the cost of outpatient versus day-case hysteroscopy. BJOG 2004;111(3):243–8.

3. Khan Z, El-Nashar SA, Hopkins MR, et al. Efficacy and safety of global endometrial ablation after cesarean delivery: a cohort study. Am J Obstet Gynecol 2011; 205(5):450.e1–4.
4. Gurtcheff SE, Sharp HT. Complications associated with global endometrial ablation: the utility of the MAUDE database. Obstet Gynecol 2003;102(6): 1278–82.
5. Rooney KE, Cholhan HJ. Vesico-uterine fistula after endometrial ablation in a woman with prior cesarean deliveries. Obstet Gynecol 2010;115(2 Pt 2):450–1.
6. Della Badia C, Nyirjesy P, Atogho A. Endometrial ablation devices: review of a manufacturer and user facility device experience database. J Minim Invasive Gynecol 2007;14(4):436–41.
7. Lethaby A, Shepperd S, Cooke I, et al. Endometrial resection and ablation versus hysterectomy for heavy menstrual bleeding. Cochrane Database Syst Rev 2000;(2):CD000329.
8. Sharp HT. Assessment of new technology in the treatment of idiopathic menorrhagia and uterine leiomyomata. Obstet Gynecol 2006;108(4):990–1003.
9. Roth TM, Rivlin ME. Tuboovarian abscess: a postoperative complication of endometrial ablation. Obstet Gynecol 2004;104(5 Pt 2):1198–9.
10. Brown J, Blank K. Minimally invasive endometrial ablation device complications and use outside of the manufacturers' instructions. Obstet Gynecol 2012; 120(4):865–70.
11. ACOG Committee on Practice Bulletins–Gynecology. ACOG practice bulletin No. 104: antibiotic prophylaxis for gynecologic procedures. Obstet Gynecol 2009; 113(5):1180–9.
12. Thinkhamrop J, Laopaiboon M, Lumbiganon P. Prophylactic antibiotics for transcervical intrauterine procedures. Cochrane Database Syst Rev 2007;(3):CD005637.
13. Sharp HT. Endometrial ablation: postoperative complications. Am J Obstet Gynecol 2012;207(4):242–7.
14. McCausland AM, McCausland VM. Long-term complications of endometrial ablation: cause, diagnosis, treatment, and prevention. J Minim Invasive Gynecol 2007;14(4):399–406.
15. Carey ET, El-Nashar SA, Hopkins MR, et al. Pathologic characteristics of hysterectomy specimens in women undergoing hysterectomy after global endometrial ablation. J Minim Invasive Gynecol 2011;18(1):96–9.
16. Townsend DE, McCausland V, McCausland A, et al. Post-ablation-tubal sterilization syndrome. Obstet Gynecol 1993;82(3):422–4.
17. McCausland AM, McCausland VM. Frequency of symptomatic cornual hematometra and postablation tubal sterilization syndrome after total rollerball endometrial ablation: a 10-year follow-up. Am J Obstet Gynecol 2002;186(6):1274–80 [discussion: 1280–3].
18. Yin CS. Pregnancy after hysteroscopic endometrial ablation without endometrial preparation: a report of five cases and a literature review. Taiwan J Obstet Gynecol 2010;49(3):311–9.
19. Lo JS, Pickersgill A. Pregnancy after endometrial ablation: English literature review and case report. J Minim Invasive Gynecol 2006;13(2):88–91.
20. AlHilli MM, Hopkins MR, Famuyide AO. Endometrial cancer after endometrial ablation: systematic review of medical literature. J Minim Invasive Gynecol 2011;18(3):393–400.
21. Daniels JP, Middleton LJ, Champaneria R, et al. Second generation endometrial ablation techniques for heavy menstrual bleeding: network meta-analysis. BMJ 2012;344:e2564.

22. Clark TJ, Samuels N, Malick S, et al. Bipolar radiofrequency compared with thermal balloon endometrial ablation in the office: a randomized controlled trial. Obstet Gynecol 2011;117(5):1228.
23. Marjoribanks J, Lethaby A, Farquhar C. Surgery versus medical therapy for heavy menstrual bleeding. Cochrane Database Syst Rev 2006;(2):CD003855.
24. Brown PM, Farquhar CM, Lethaby A, et al. Cost-effectiveness analysis of levonorgestrel intrauterine system and thermal balloon ablation for heavy menstrual bleeding. BJOG 2006;113(7):797–803.
25. Comino R, Torrejon R. Hysterectomy after endometrial ablation-resection. J Am Assoc Gynecol Laparosc 2004;11(4):495–9.
26. A randomised trial of endometrial ablation versus hysterectomy for the treatment of dysfunctional uterine bleeding: outcome at four years. Aberdeen Endometrial Ablation Trials Group. Br J Obstet Gynaecol 1999;106(4):360–6.
27. Roberts TE, Tsourapas A, Middleton LJ, et al. Hysterectomy, endometrial ablation, and levonorgestrel releasing intrauterine system (Mirena) for treatment of heavy menstrual bleeding: cost effectiveness analysis. BMJ 2011;342:d2202.
28. El-Nashar SA, Hopkins MR, Creedon DJ, et al. Prediction of treatment outcomes after global endometrial ablation. Obstet Gynecol 2009;113(1):97–106.
29. Gangadharan A, Revel A, Shushan A. Endometrial thermal balloon ablation in women with previous cesarean delivery: pilot study. J Minim Invasive Gynecol 2010;17:358.
30. Endometrial ablation, ACOG practice bulletin No. 81. Obstet Gynecol 2007;109:1233–48.

Contraceptive Procedures

Anitra Beasley, MD, MPH*, Ann Schutt-Ainé, MD

KEYWORDS

- Intrauterine device • Contraceptive implant • Levonorgestrel • Etonogestrel

KEY POINTS

- Long-acting reversible contraceptives (LARCs), such as intrauterine devices (IUDs), and implants, are among the most effective forms of contraception available. There are few contraindications to their use, and insertion and removal are straightforward procedures that are well tolerated in the outpatient office setting.
- The American College of Obstetrician and Gynecologists recognizes high upfront patient costs as a barrier to LARC use and advocates for coverage of all contraceptive methods by all insurance plans.
- In July 2011, the Institute of Medicine published an expert committee report on preventative services for women that should be considered in developing comprehensive health guidelines. It defined preventative services as "measures—including medications, procedures, devices, tests, education, and counseling—shown to improve well-being and/or decrease the likelihood or delay the onset of a targeted disease or condition."
- Among these services are the full range of US Food and Drug Administration-approved contraceptive devices. In August 2011, the Department of Health and Human Services incorporated these recommendations into preventative services covered by health plans under the Patient Protection and Affordable Care Act (ACA), without cost sharing by the patient.
- Although there are continuing legal battles over the ACA, it is hoped that with its full implementation over the coming years, women will have increased access to these safe, effective forms of birth control.

Although most women desire to control the size and spacing of their family, the rate of unintended pregnancy in the United States remains high. Approximately half of all pregnancies are unintended,[1] which is significantly higher than in many other developed countries.[2] Reducing unintended pregnancy is a national public health goal. The US Department of Health and Human Services' Healthy People 2020 campaign aims to reduce the rate of unintended pregnancy by 10% over the next several years,[3] and increased use of long-acting reversible contraceptives (LARCs) (intrauterine

Department of Obstetrics & Gynecology, Baylor College of Medicine, One Baylor Plaza, MS-610, Houston, TX 77030, USA
* Corresponding author.
E-mail address: anitra.beasley@bcm.edu

Obstet Gynecol Clin N Am 40 (2013) 697–729
http://dx.doi.org/10.1016/j.ogc.2013.08.003 obgyn.theclinics.com
0889-8545/13/$ – see front matter

devices and implants) can help meet this goal. Fortunately the uptake of LARC devices is increasing, with almost 8% of women using an intrauterine device (IUD) and 1% using an implant.[4]

This article will cover indications and contraindications for IUD and implant use, techniques for insertion and removal, and management of complications.

INTRAUTERINE DEVICES

Multiple IUDs are used throughout the world, but only 3 intrauterine devices are available in the United States: the Copper 380A (ParaGard, Teva Woman's Health Inc., North Wales, Pennsylvania), a 13.5 mg levonorgestrel (LNG)-releasing system (Skyla, Bayer, Pittsburgh, Pennsylvania), and the 52 mg LNG-releasing system (Mirena, Bayer).

COPPER T 380A (TCU-380A) IUD

The TCu-380A is a T-shaped, 36 mm × 32 mm polyethylene device impregnated with barium sulfate to increase radiograph visibility. Copper wire is wound around the vertical stem, and the arms have tubular copper sleeves. A monofilament string is tied to the bottom of the stem to aid in device removal. The TCu-380A is highly effective, with a failure rate of 0.8% at 1 year.[5]

LNG INTRAUTERINE SYSTEMS

The LNG intrauterine systems are also T-shaped, barium-impregnated polyethylene devices with monofilament threads at the base; however, both devices contain a steroid reservoir that delivers LNG mainly to the endometrium and surrounding tissues. The 13.5 mg system (LNG-14) is 28 × 30 mm and initially releases approximately 14 μg LNG per day, which declines to 5 μg/d after 3 years.[6] The 52 mg system (LNG-20) is 32 × 32 mm and initially releases 20 μg of LNG per day; this rate is reduced by approximately 50% after 5 years.[7] Both devices are highly effective, with a failure rate of approximately 0.2% for Mirena[5] and 0.4% for Skyla.[6]

INDICATIONS/CONTRAINDICATIONS

Intrauterine devices are US Food and Drug Administration (FDA) approved for intrauterine contraception for 3 to 10 years, depending on the device. The ParaGard is approved for up to 10 years of continuous use and the Mirena for up to 5 years, but data demonstrate reasonable effectiveness as long as 12 and 7 years, respectively.[8–12] Skyla earned FDA approval in early 2013 and is indicated for the prevention of pregnancy for up to 3 years. Additionally, the copper IUD may be inserted as emergency contraception within 5 days of unprotected intercourse and may be left in for ongoing pregnancy prevention.[13] The effectiveness of using an LNG-releasing IUD for emergency contraception has not been studied and therefore is not recommended.

Mirena is also indicated for treatment of heavy menstrual bleeding for women who choose to use intrauterine contraception as their method for pregnancy prevention. Although off-label, it has been used for medical management of women with endometrial hyperplasia who desire to retain fertility or are poor surgical candidates.[14] Postmenopausal women on estrogen-containing hormone replacement therapy have also used this device for endometrial protection.

Although FDA labeling of contraceptives is often more restrictive than evidence-based guidance, there are few actual contraindications to IUD use. The World Health

Organization (WHO) publishes medical eligibility criteria for contraceptive use, which use systematic reviews of medical and epidemiologic research to develop evidence-based guidelines for specific contraceptive methods and medical conditions. These have been adapted by the Centers for Disease Control and Prevention (CDC) to produce the US Medical Eligibility Criteria for Contraceptive Use (USMEC). An explanation of the classification categories is in **Box 1**.

Although Mirena labeling still recommends use in multiparous women, such restrictions have been removed from the ParaGard labeling. Additional restrictions, including previous recommendations for use only by women in stable, mutually monogamous relationships and without a history of pelvic inflammatory disease or ectopic pregnancy, have also been removed, and—despite package labeling—evidence supports similar, more liberal use with the Mirena. **Tables 1** and **2** show the contraindications to the copper and LNG IUDs described in the FDA-approved prescribing information, as well as the classification of each contraindication in the USMEC[15] and WHO Medical Eligibility for Contraceptive Use.[16] The WHO and USMEC do not specifically address Skyla, as they were last updated prior to its introduction.

INSERTION AND REMOVAL

Preprocedure counseling should take place prior to IUD insertion. Generally, all indicated and appropriate methods of reversible and permanent contraception are discussed. Once a patient has elected for IUD use, more specific risks are reviewed, including infection, uterine perforation, irregular bleeding, and failure. It is important to note that while IUD use decreases the risk of ectopic pregnancy overall, there is actually an increased risk of ectopic pregnancy with IUD failures. Each IUD is ultimately associated with a unique bleeding pattern, as previously discussed; however, all patients should expect unscheduled bleeding for 3 to 6 months after insertion.

Although manufacturer instructions vary, IUDs can be inserted at any time during the menstrual cycle as long as there is reasonable certainty that the patient is not pregnant. Two negative pregnancy tests are not necessary prior to IUD placement and, in fact, do not actually decrease the risk of pregnancy at the time of IUD insertion. In patients with a low risk for current chlamydial or gonorrheal infection, there is no need for preprocedure sexually transmitted infection (STI) testing. If desired, testing can be done at the time of insertion and if necessary, and STIs can be treated later without immediate removal of the IUD. There is no benefit for the common practice of inserting the IUD only during menses.[17] IUDs also can be inserted immediately after vaginal or cesarean delivery or after abortion without increased risk of infection, uterine perforation, bleeding, or uterine subinvolution.[16,18] Insertion should be avoided if there is any increased risk or evidence of intrauterine infection.[18,19] Expulsion rates are lowest when insertion occurs within 10 minutes of placental delivery.[18,20] In addition,

Box 1
Classification categories for US and WHO medical eligibility criteria

1. A condition for which there is no restriction for the use of method
2. A condition for which the advantages of use generally outweigh the theoretical or proven risks
3. A condition for which the theoretical or proven risks usually outweigh the advantages of use
4. A condition that represents an unacceptable health risk if the method is used

Table 1
Contraindications to TCu-380A IUD use

Contraindication Per Package Labeling	USMEC and WHO Category		Comment
Known or suspected pregnancy	4		The IUD is not indicated during pregnancy and should not be used because of the risk for serious pelvic infection and septic spontaneous abortion
Uterine abnormalities resulting in distortion of the cavity	4		An abnormality that distorts the uterine cavity might preclude proper IUD placement
Acute pelvic inflammatory disease	Initiation 4	Continuation 2	—
Postpartum or postabortal endometritis within the last 3 mo	4		Immediate insertion following puerperal sepsis or septic abortion might substantially worsen the condition
Known or suspected uterine or cervical malignancy	Initiation 4	Continuation 2	—
Genital bleeding of unknown etiology	Initiation 4	Continuation 2	—
Mucopurulent cervicitis	Initiation 4	Continuation 2	—
Allergy to any component of the IUD	N/A		—
Wilson disease	N/A		—
A previously placed IUD that has not been removed	N/A		—

placement at the time of cesarean deliveries has lower expulsion rates than does post-placental vaginal insertions.[20]

The insertion techniques differ for each of the intrauterine devices; however, a pelvic examination should be performed to establish the size and position of the uterus prior to any IUD placement. Prescribing instructions call for cleaning the cervix and the vagina with an aseptic solution, and most practitioners do; however, no evidence supports this practice.[21] A tenaculum should be applied to the cervix and gentle traction used to align the cervical canal and the uterus. This will facilitate fundal placement; the uterus also may be sounded to better gauge the length of the uterus.

ParaGard

ParaGard is packaged together with an insertion tube and solid white rod in a sterilized pouch. A movable flange on the insertion tube aids in gauging the depth of insertion (**Fig. 1**).

To use ParaGard, open the package and sterilely load the device into the insertion tube no more than 5 minutes prior placement by folding the horizontal arms against the stem and pushing the tips gently into the inserter tube. If sterile gloves are not available, this step can be accomplished while the IUD is still in the package (**Fig. 2**).

Table 2
Contraindications to LNG IUD use

Contraindication Per Package Labeling	USMEC and WHO Category		Comment
Known or suspected pregnancy	4		The IUD is not indicated during pregnancy and should not be used because of the risk for serious pelvic infection and septic spontaneous abortion
Abnormalities of the uterus resulting in distortion of the uterine cavity	4		An abnormality that distorts the uterine cavity might preclude proper IUD placement
Acute pelvic inflammatory disease (PID)	Initiation 4	Continuation 2	—
History of PID unless there has been a subsequent intrauterine pregnancy	1 if past PID, with subsequent pregnancy 2 if past PID, without subsequent pregnancy		IUDs do not protect against STI/HIV/PID; in women at low risk for STIs, IUD insertion poses little risk for PID; current risk for STIs and desire for future pregnancy are relevant considerations
Postpartum or postabortal endometritis within the last 3 mo	4		Immediate insertion following puerperal sepsis or septic abortion might substantially worsen the condition
Known or suspected uterine or cervical neoplasia	Initiation 4	Continuation 2	—
Known or suspected breast cancer or other progestin-sensitive tumor	3 if past cancer and no evidence of current disease for 5 y 4 if current cancer		—
Genital or uterine bleeding of unknown etiology	Initiation 4	Continuation 2	—
Untreated active cervicitis	Initiation 4	Continuation 2	—
Untreated vaginitis or other lower genital tract infections	2		—
Hypersensitivity to any component of the IUD	N/A		—
A previously placed IUD that has not been removed	N/A		—
Increased susceptibility to pelvic infection (Mirena only)	Initiation 2/3	Continuation 2	The condition is a Category 3 if there is a very high individual likelihood of exposure to gonorrhea or chlamydia

Next, the solid white rod should be introduced into the distal end of the insertion tube until it touches the bottom of the device. The blue flange should be adjusted to the sounded depth of the uterus and the flange rotated so that the horizontal arms of the T and the long axis of the flange are in the same horizontal plane. The loaded

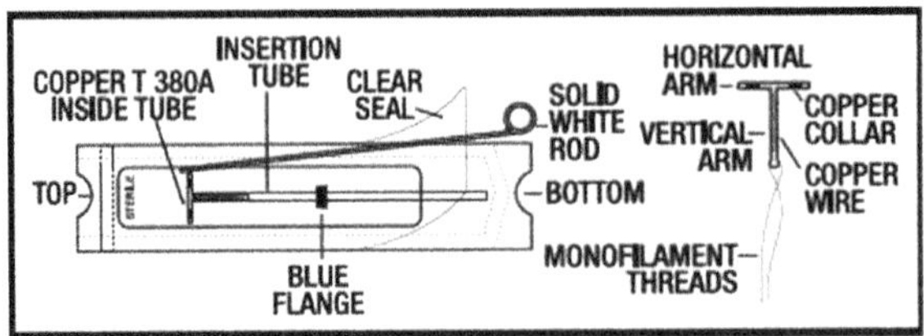

Fig. 1. ParaGard is packaged together with an insertion tube and solid white rod in a sterilized pouch. A movable flange on the insertion tube aids in gauging the depth of insertion. (*Courtesy of* Teva Women's Health.)

insertion tube should be passed through the cervical canal until the device touches the fundus (**Fig. 3**).

The arms of the device should be released by holding the rod steady and pulling back on the insertion tube (**Fig. 4**). The insertion tube should be carefully pushed upwards to the fundus until slight resistance is felt (**Fig. 5**). The insertion rod and then the tube should be withdrawn (**Fig. 6**). Finally, the strings should be trimmed to 3 to 4 cm outside the cervix (**Fig. 7**).

Skyla

Skyla is supplied within an inserter in sterile packaging. The inserter consists of a 2-sided body that is integrated with a prebent insertion tube, flange, and slider (**Fig. 8**).

To insert Skyla, open the package. Lift the handle of the inserter and remove it from the sterile package. The prescribing information calls for the use of sterile gloves. However, the design of the inserter obviates the need for direct handling of the part of the inserter that will be placed inside of the uterus or the IUD itself. Therefore nonsterile gloves may be used (**Fig. 9**).

Next one should push the slider forward (in the direction of the arrow) as far as possible to load the device into the insertion tube (**Fig. 10**). Maintain pressure on the slider in the forward position, as once released, Skyla cannot be reloaded.

The upper edge of the flange should be adjusted sterilely to the corresponding uterine depth (**Fig. 11**). The inserter should be advanced through the cervix until the flange is approximately 1.5 to 2 cm from the cervix (**Fig. 12**). The slider should be moved down to the mark to release the arms (**Fig. 13**).

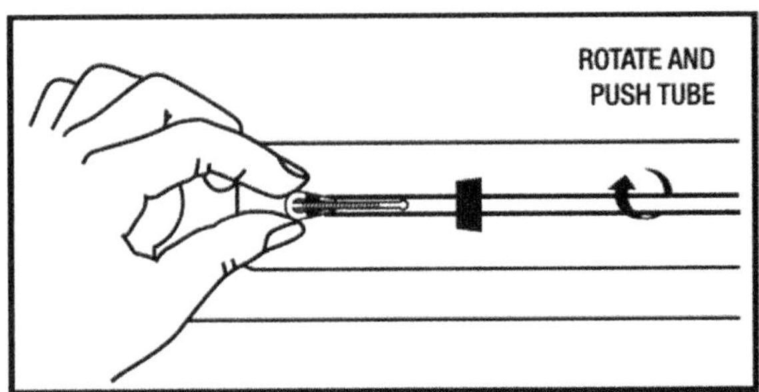

Fig. 2. The package should be opened and the device sterilely loaded into the insertion tube no more than 5 minutes prior placement by folding the horizontal arms against the stem and pushing the tips gently into the inserter tube. (*Courtesy of* Teva Women's Health.)

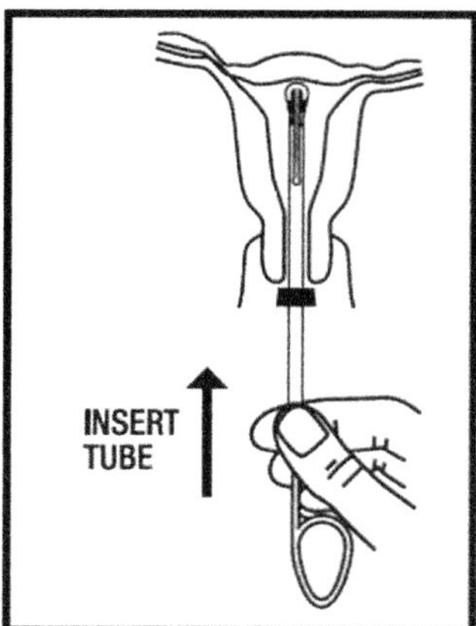

Fig. 3. The loaded insertion tube should be passed through the cervical canal until the device touches the fundus. (*Courtesy of* Teva Women's Health.)

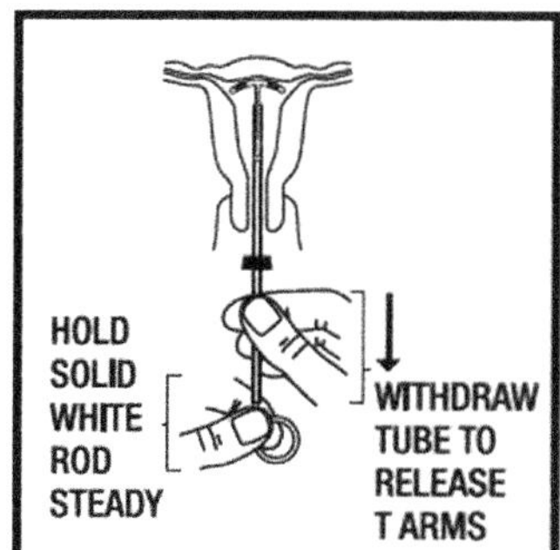

Fig. 4. The arms of the device should be released by holding the rod steady and pulling back on the insertion tube. (*Courtesy of* Teva Women's Health.)

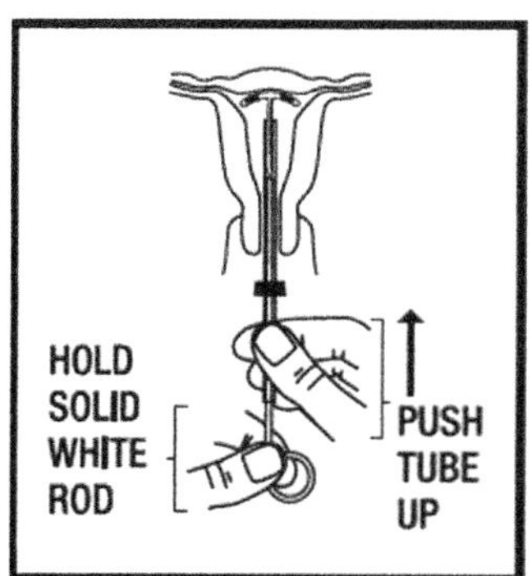

Fig. 5. One should carefully push the insertion tube upwards to the fundus until slight resistance is felt. (*Courtesy of* Teva Women's Health.)

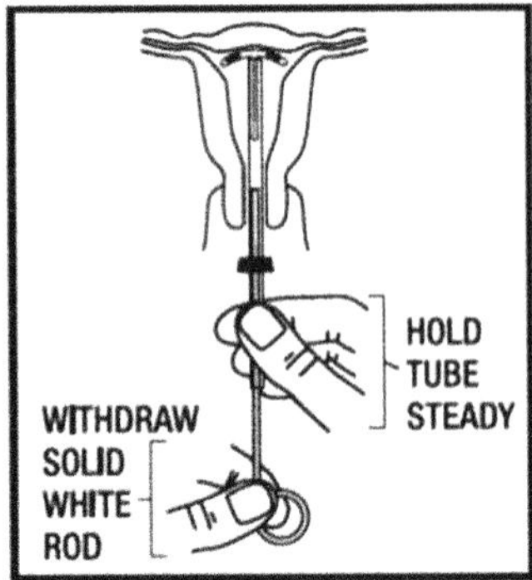

Fig. 6. The insertion rod and then the tube should be withdrawn. (*Courtesy of* Teva Women's Health.)

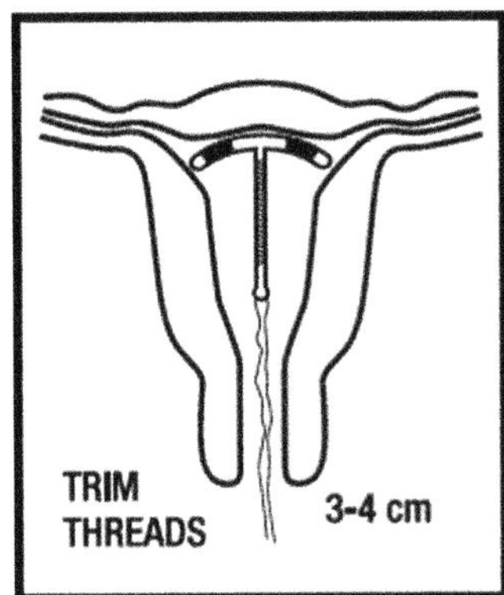

Fig. 7. The strings should be trimmed to 3–4 cm outside the cervix. (*Courtesy of* Teva Women's Health.)

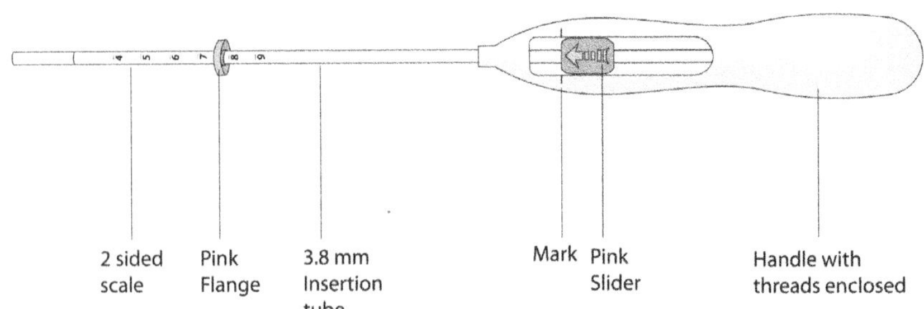

Fig. 8. Skyla is supplied within an inserter in sterile packaging. The inserter consists of a 2-sided body that is integrated with a prebent insertion tube, flange, and slider. (*Courtesy of* Bayer HealthCare Pharmaceuticals Inc.)

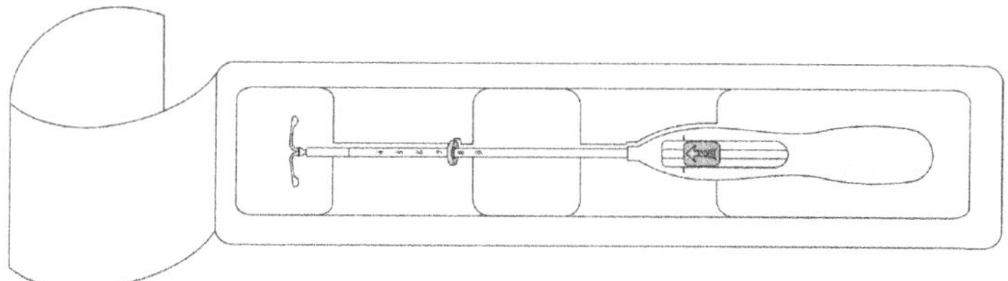

Fig. 9. The package should be opened. The handle of the inserter should be lifted and removed from the sterile package. The prescribing information calls for the use of sterile gloves. However, the design of the inserter obviates the need for direct handling of the part of the inserter that will be placed inside of the uterus or the IUD itself. Therefore non-sterile gloves may be used. (*Courtesy of* Bayer HealthCare Pharmaceuticals Inc.)

The inserter should be advanced gently toward the fundus (**Fig. 14**). The device should be released from the inserter by moving the slider all the way down (**Fig. 15**). Finally, the inserter should be withdrawn from the uterus, and the treads should be trimmed to approximately 3 cm from the cervix (**Fig. 16**).

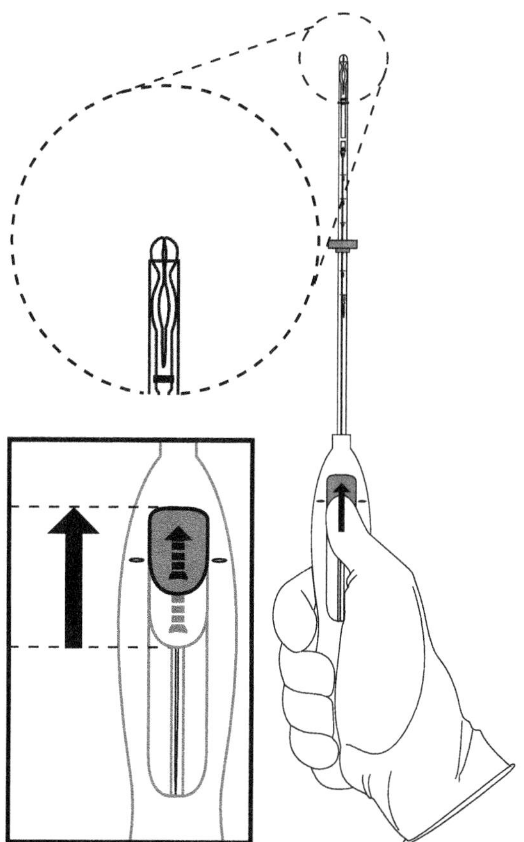

Fig. 10. The slider should be pushed forward (in the direction of the *arrow*) as far as possible to load the device into the insertion tube. (*Courtesy of* Bayer HealthCare Pharmaceuticals Inc.)

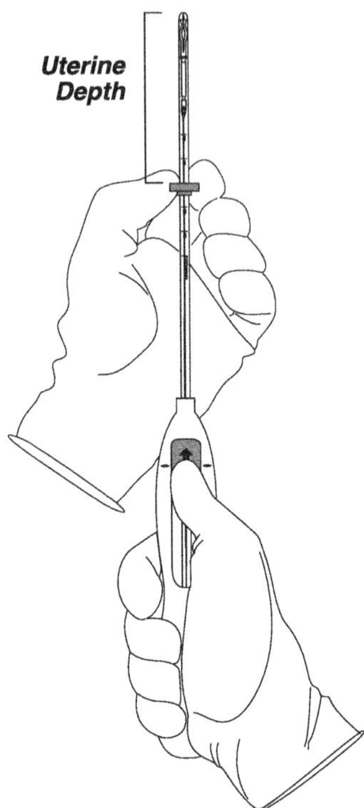

Fig. 11. One should sterilely adjust the upper edge of the flange to the corresponding uterine depth. (*Courtesy of* Bayer HealthCare Pharmaceuticals Inc.)

Mirena

Mirena is supplied within an inserter in sterile packaging. The inserter consists of a 2-sided body that is integrated with a prebent insertion tube, flange, slider, and string lock (**Fig. 17**).

To use Mirena, one should lift the handle of the inserter and remove it from the sterile package. The prescribing information calls for the use of sterile gloves. However, the design of the inserter obviates the need for direct handling of the part of the inserter that will be placed inside of the uterus or the IUD itself. Therefore nonsterile gloves may be used. The strings should be carefully released so that they hang free.

A thumb or forefinger should be placed on the slider, ensuring that it is in the position at the top of the handle. With the arms in a horizontal position, both threads should be pulled to load the device into the insertion tube (**Fig. 18**).

The threads in the cleft at the bottom of the handle should be secured. The upper edge of the flange should be sterilely adjusted to the corresponding uterine depth. Pressure on the slider should be maintained in the forward position.

The inserter should be advanced through the cervix until the flange is approximately 1.5 to 2 cm from the cervix (**Fig. 19**). The slider should be moved down to the mark to release the arms (**Figs. 20** and **21**). The inserter should be advanced gently toward the fundus while, holding the slider in its current position (**Fig. 22**).

The device should be released from the inserter by moving the slider all the way down (**Fig. 23**). Finally, the inserter should be withdrawn from the uterus, and the treads should be trimmed (**Fig. 24**).

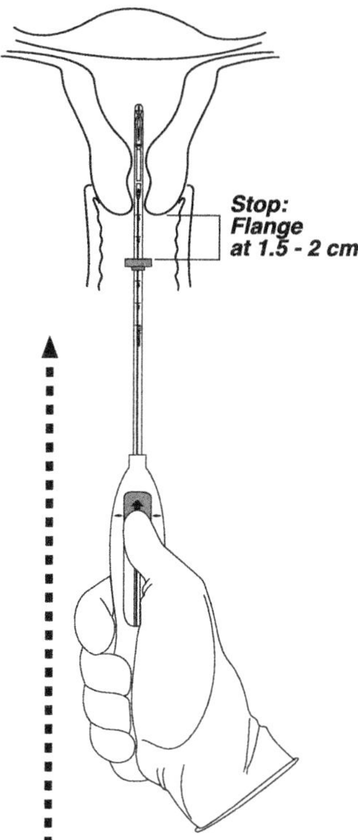

Fig. 12. The inserter should be advanced through the cervix until the flange is approximately 1.5–2 cm from the cervix. (*Courtesy of* Bayer HealthCare Pharmaceuticals Inc.)

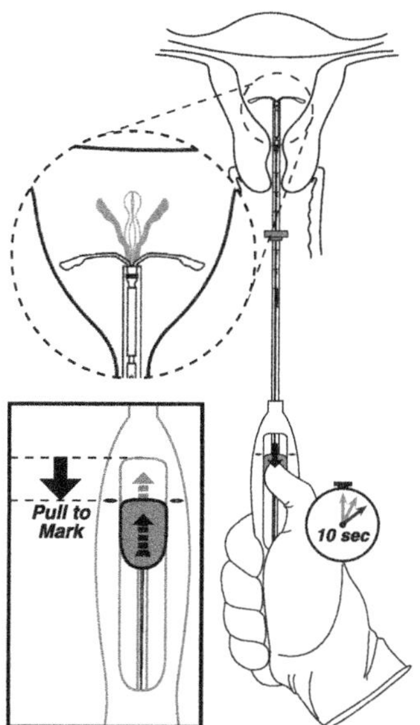

Fig. 13. The slider should be moved down to the mark to release the arms. (*Courtesy of* Bayer HealthCare Pharmaceuticals Inc.)

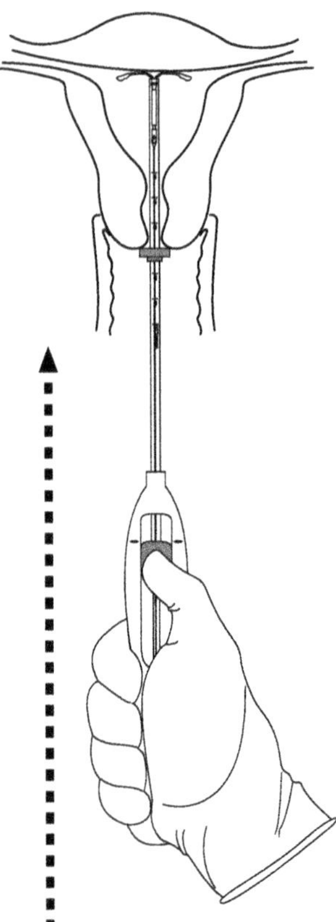

Fig. 14. The inserter should be advanced gently toward the fundus. (*Courtesy of* Bayer HealthCare Pharmaceuticals Inc.)

If poor placement is suspected with any of the devices, placement should be checked with an ultrasound. If the IUD is not placed correctly, it should be removed and a new device inserted. All IUDs may be removed at any time by gently pulling on the exposed strings with forceps.

COMPLICATIONS AND MANAGEMENT

Cramping and Pain

Discomfort may be felt at the time of IUD insertion and may be followed by cramping and pain over the next several minutes. Prophylactic administration of nonsteroidal anti-inflammatory drugs (NSAIDs) or administration of a paracervical block generally has not been found to be helpful.[22,23] More recent studies have found that intrauterine or intracervical anesthesia also does not decrease pain scores.[24–26] However, preprocedure misoprostol may increase the ease of placement when a difficult insertion is anticipated, such as in nuliparous women or those with cervical stenosis. A paracervical block may be useful in women who require cervical dilation to facilitate placement. Manipulation of the cervix and the cervical os can occasionally result in vasovagal reactions. The patient should remain supine, but once she feels well, she can be discharged from clinic. Severe pain or pain that develops later may reflect

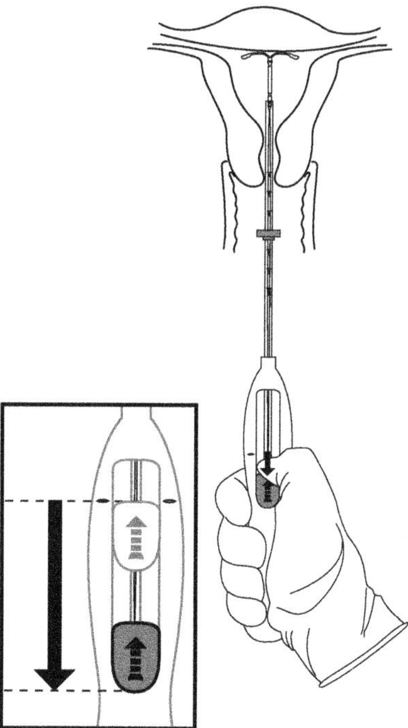

Fig. 15. The device should be released from the inserter by moving the slider all the way down. (*Courtesy of* Bayer HealthCare Pharmaceuticals Inc.)

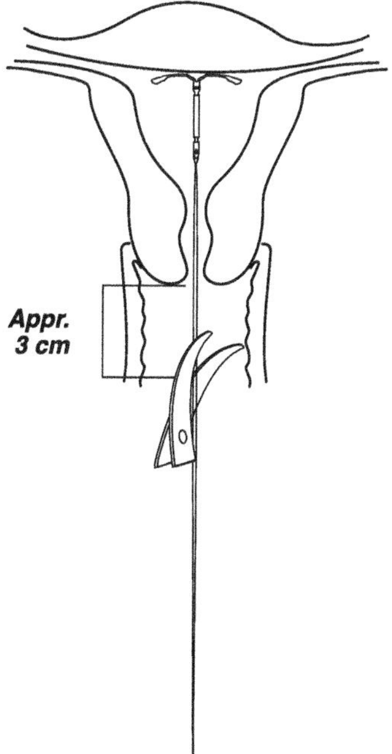

Fig. 16. One should withdraw the inserter from the uterus and trim the treads to approximately 3 cm from the cervix. (*Courtesy of* Bayer HealthCare Pharmaceuticals Inc.)

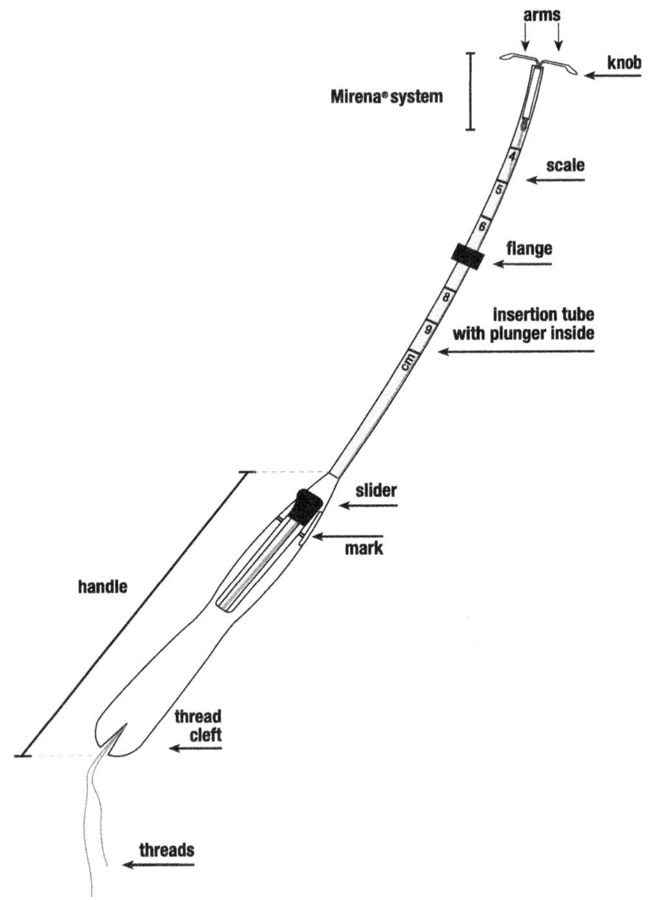

Fig. 17. Mirena is supplied within an inserter in sterile packaging. The inserter consists of a 2-sided body that is integrated with a prebent insertion tube, flange, slider, and string lock. (*Courtesy of* Bayer HealthCare Pharmaceuticals Inc.)

threatened or partial expulsion, dislodgement, infection, or pregnancy, and should be investigated.

Perforation

Although it may not be detected until later, perforation of the uterus occurs at a rate of less than 0.1%.[27] Perforation at the time of procedure may be suspected when instruments pass further than expected, often without a discernable loss of resistance, or if the patient experiences sudden or unexpected pain. If perforation with the uterine sound is suspected, the patient may simply be observed, and as long as there are no symptoms of intraabdominal bleeding, she may be sent home. If perforation occurs with the IUD, the device should be removed, if possible, by gently tugging on the strings.

Traditionally, prompt removal of copper-containing IUDs by laparotomy or laparoscopy was recommended in the case of uterine perforations unrecognized at the time of placement, as copper can induce adhesion formation, which may involve the omentum, adnexa, or bowel. In contrast, nonmedicated and LNG-releasing devices do not

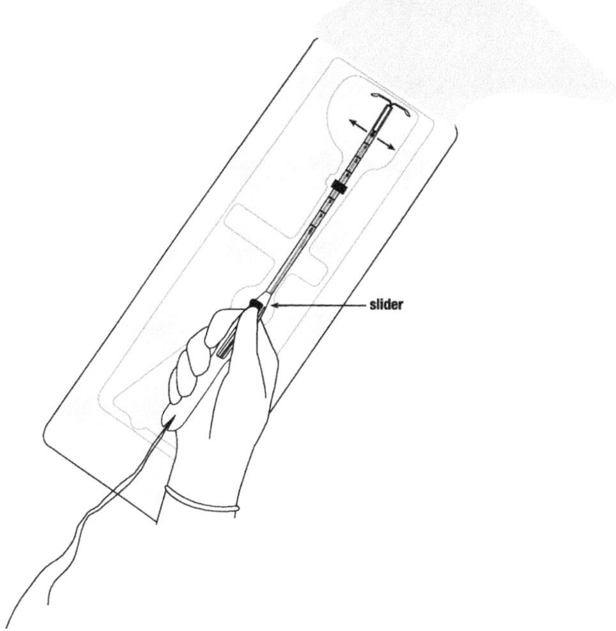

Fig. 18. A thumb or forefinger should be placed on the slider, ensuring that it is in the position at the top of the handle. With the arms in a horizontal position, both threads should be pulled to load the device into the insertion tube. (*Courtesy of* Bayer HealthCare Pharmaceuticals Inc.)

provoke such reactions but were nonetheless often removed. Recent evidence has called into question the need to remove intraperitoneally displaced devices in asymptomatic patients.[28,29] All women should use an alternate form of contraception, as extrauterine IUDs, including the LNG devices, provide less than ideal protection from pregnancy.[30]

Follow-up

Many providers plan for a follow-up visit after the patient's next menses. Although a routine postprocedure visit is not required, this visit can be used to confirm that the IUD is still in place and that there are no signs of infection. More importantly, the visit can be helpful in reassuring women experiencing adverse effects who are considering discontinuation of the IUD. If a routine follow-up visit is not scheduled, women should be encouraged to return at any time if they have problems, questions, or concerns, in particular, if they have previously felt the IUD strings and now cannot; the strings seem too long; or the IUD is palpable.

Irregular Bleeding

Adverse effects of all IUDs include menstrual irregularities. Irregular bleeding is common up to 3 to 6 months following insertion, regardless of device type. With time, the bleeding profiles will differ between the 2 devices; heavier bleeding is more common with the TCu-380A, and unscheduled bleeding is more common with the LNG systems. Excessive bleeding and dysmenorrhea associated with the copper IUD usually normalizes but can be treated with NSAIDs. With Mirena, approximately 20% of

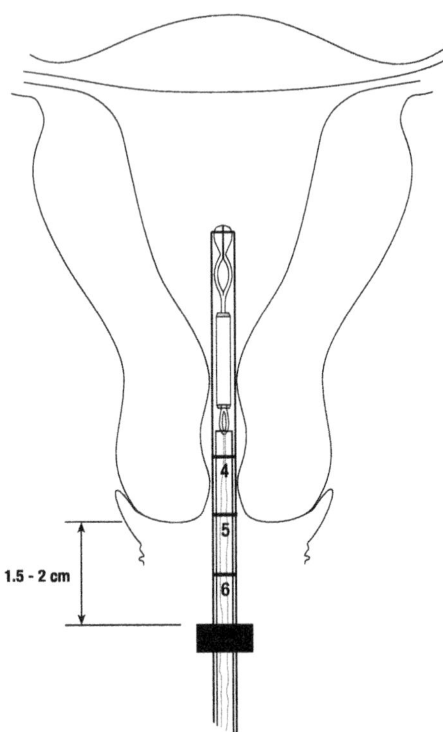

Fig. 19. The inserter should be advanced through the cervix until the flange is approximately 1.5–2 cm from the cervix. (*Courtesy of* Bayer HealthCare Pharmaceuticals Inc.)

women become amenorrheic within 1 year, and most others will experience shorter, lighter cycles.[7] Amenorrhea develops by the end of the first year of use in only 6% of Skyla users. In studies, 20% experienced infrequent bleeding, 8% frequent bleeding, 9% prolonged bleeding, and 23% more irregular bleeding.[6]

Expulsion

Two percent to 10% of IUD users spontaneously expel their IUD within the first year.[31] Expulsions may be silent or can be associated with unusual vaginal discharge, cramping, pain, spotting, dyspareunia, absence or lengthening of the IUD string, or presence of the hard plastic at the cervical os or in the vagina. Younger age, nulliparity, menorrhagia, and severe dysmenorrhea are risk factors for expulsion.[31,32]

String Problems

Missing strings may signal an unsuspected perforation, spontaneous expulsion, or simply migration of the strings into the cervical canal or endometrial cavity. Ultrasound should be used to confirm the location of the device. However, if a patient desires to continue IUD use, missing string should not be considered an indication for removal once proper intrauterine placement has been confirmed. When the device is not seen on ultrasound, an abdominal radiogram should be performed to determine if the device is in the abdomen/pelvis or has been expelled.

If the device is in the uterus, and the patient desires removal, a cytobrush may be used to tease the strings out of the cervix; narrow forceps, such as Alligator forceps

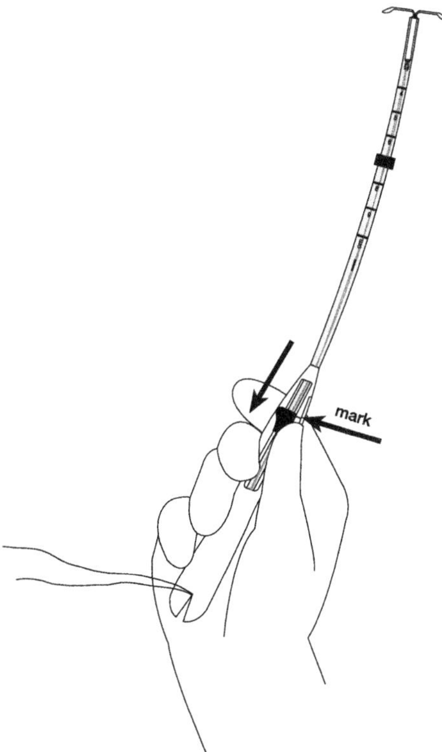

Fig. 20. The slider should be moved down to the mark to release the arms. (*Courtesy of* Bayer HealthCare Pharmaceuticals Inc.)

(**Fig. 25**), may be used to grasp strings within the cervical canal or remove the IUD from the uterine cavity. Ultrasound guidance and cervical dilation may be helpful. When engaging in more invasive procedures, a paracervical block should be used. If removal is unsuccessful, hysteroscopy may be of benefit.

If the patient's partner complains of discomfort during intercourse, the strings may be too short or too long. If the strings are too short, they may be cut even shorter so that they rest in the endocervical canal. If they are too long, they may either be wrapped around the cervix or cut to a shorter length. If the strings become longer with time, check for partial expulsion.

Pregnancy

Women who become pregnant while using an IUD should be evaluated for ectopic pregnancy. A pregnancy that occurs with an IUD in place is more likely to be ectopic than a pregnancy in the general population. However, because IUDs prevent most pregnancies, women who use IUDs have a lower risk of ectopic pregnancy than women who use less effective or no contraception.

If an intrauterine pregnancy occurs with an IUD in place and the string is visible, the IUD should be removed, regardless of plans for the pregnancy. Early removal reduces, but does not eliminate, the risk of spontaneous abortion, premature delivery, septic abortion, and chorioamnionitis.[33] Removal is usually inadvisable if the strings are not visible and the patient desires to continue the pregnancy; removal under these

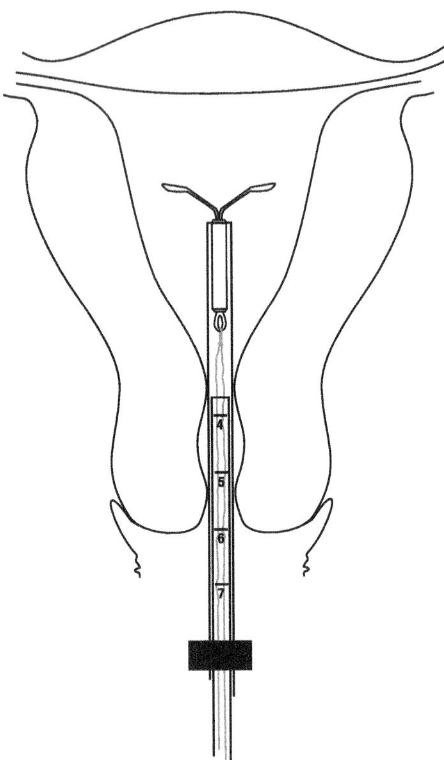

Fig. 21. The slider should be moved down to the mark to release the arms. (*Courtesy of* Bayer HealthCare Pharmaceuticals Inc.)

circumstances is considered more controversial as there seems to be a greater risk to disrupt a desired pregnancy. There is no evidence of teratogenicity with fetal exposure to copper or LNG from an IUD that remains in situ.[31]

Infection

Pelvic inflammatory disease is uncommon in women using IUDs, but there is a higher risk of infection in the first 20 days following insertion.[34] Evidence is insufficient to recommend removal of IUDs in women diagnosed with acute upper genital tract infection[15]; however infections that develop after insertion should be treated and followed closely; the CDC published recommendations for treatment of upper genital tract infections.[35] Antibiotic prophylaxis should not routinely be used at insertion.[36]

Actinomyces-like Organisms on Papanicolaou Smear

Pelvic actinomycosis is an exceedingly rare but serious infection. The *Actinomyces* species is a part of the normal vaginal flora, and the presence of *Actinomyces*-like organisms on Papanicolaou smear does not predict clinical illness. An asymptomatic IUD user who has *Actinomyces*-like organisms reported on Papanicolaou smear should be informed, and nothing else needs to be done. If she has signs or symptoms of pelvic inflammatory disease, such as abdominal pain or fever, she should be treated with oral antibiotics, as *Actinomyces* species are sensitive to a variety of antibiotics, including penicillin. The device should be removed.[37]

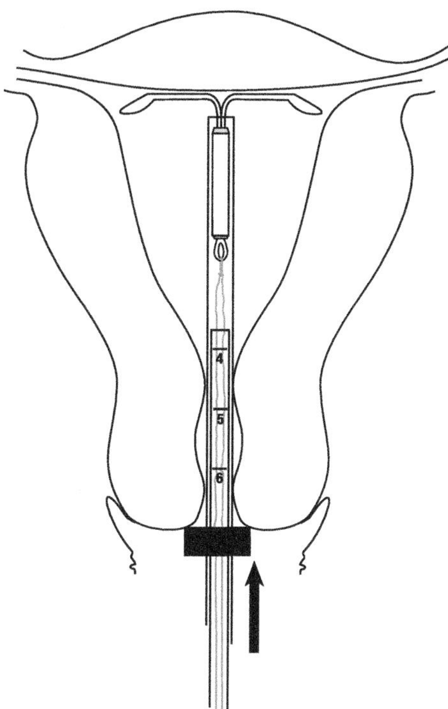

Fig. 22. The inserter should be advanced gently toward the fundus while holding the slider in its current position. (*Courtesy of* Bayer HealthCare Pharmaceuticals Inc.)

OUTCOMES

IUDs are extremely effective contraceptives, and both ParaGard and Mirena have high continuation rates. Seventy-eight percent of women were reported to be still using the ParaGard after 1 year, and 80% were reported to be still using Mirena.[5] Postmarketing experience with Skyla is limited, but in clinical trials (n = 1432), 21.9% of women discontinued use because of an adverse event. The most common adverse reactions were vulvovaginitis (20.2%), abdominal/pelvic pain (18.9%), acne/seborrhea (15.0%), ovarian cyst (13.2%), headache (12.4%), dysmenorrhea (8.6%), breast pain/discomfort (8.6%), increased bleeding (7.8%), and nausea.[6]

CONTRACEPTIVE IMPLANTS

Contraceptive implants are progestin-containing rods designed for subdermal placement, which provide long-acting reversible contraception. The etonogestrel implant (Implanon, Nexplanon, Merck & Co., Whitehouse Station, New Jersey) is currently the only available implant in the United States. Implanon was FDA approved in 2006, but beginning in 2011 has been phased out with the introduction of Nexplanon. Both are soft, flexible implants 2 mm in diameter and 4 cm in length and contain 68 mg of etonogestrel.[38] Nexplanon also contains a small amount of barium sulfate, and has been found to be bioequivalent to Implanon in situ with the advantage of clear visibility on radiograph imaging.[39] Both have similar contraceptive efficacy[40] with a typical use pregnancy rate of 0.05%.[5]

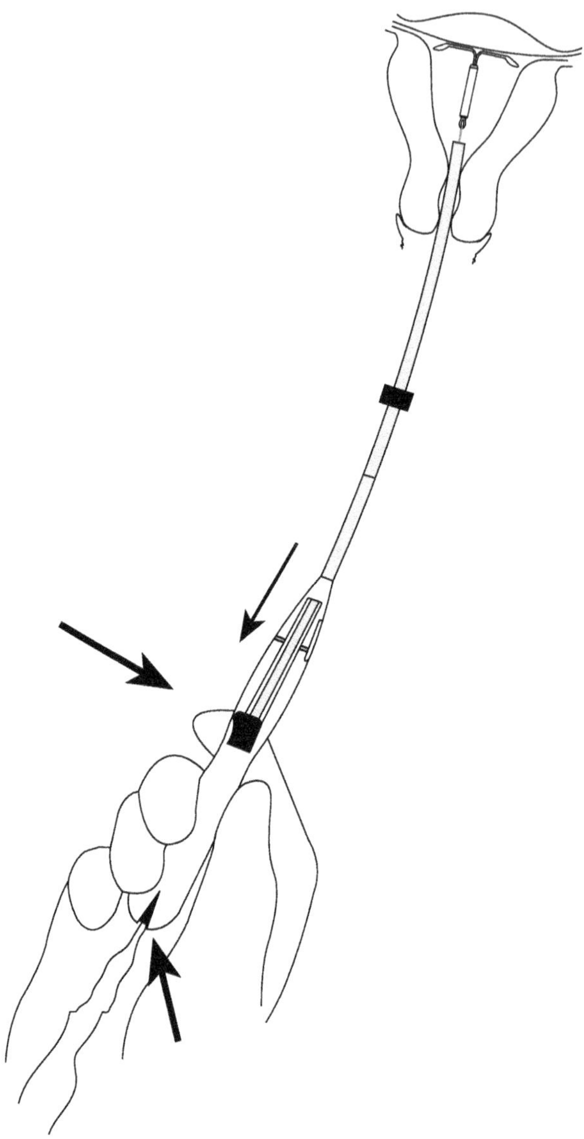

Fig. 23. The device should be released from the inserter by moving the slider all the way down. (*Courtesy of* Bayer HealthCare Pharmaceuticals Inc.)

INDICATIONS/CONTRAINDICATIONS

The etonogestrel implant is FDA approved for the prevention of pregnancy for up to 3 years.[38] However, pharmacokinetic data and studies of small numbers of women using Implanon for longer than 3 years suggest it may be effective longer.[41] **Table 3** shows the contraindications to etonogestrel implant use described in the FDA-approved prescribing information, as well as the classification of each contraindication in the USMEC[15] and WHO Medical Eligibility for Contraceptive Use.[16]

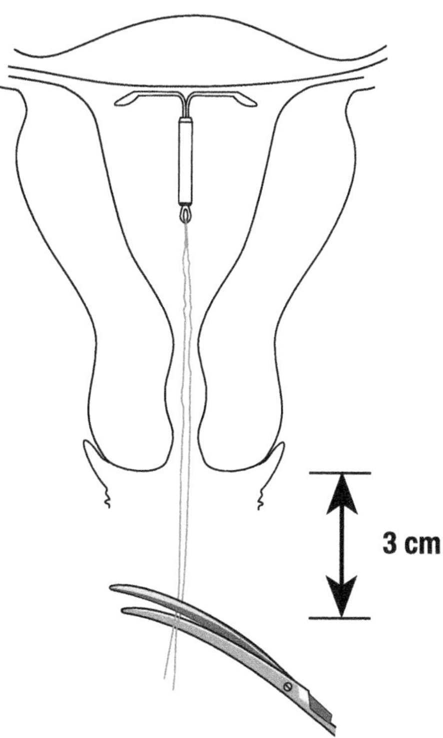

Fig. 24. One should withdraw the inserter from the uterus and trim the treads. (*Courtesy of* Bayer HealthCare Pharmaceuticals Inc.)

Preprocedure counseling and consent are important components of all office procedures, and these begin with a thorough review of all contraceptive options. Specific counseling points for the contraceptive implant should include efficacy, duration of use, return to fertility, and bleeding pattern. The typical-use failure rate for the etonogestrel implant is 0.05%,[5] making it among the most effective forms of reversible contraception available, and return to fertility is prompt, with 94% of women ovulating within 3 months, and most within 3 weeks.[41] Approximately 20% of women will have irregular bleeding while using the contraceptive implant, and another 20% will experience amenorrhea.[38] Changes in bleeding pattern are the most common reason for

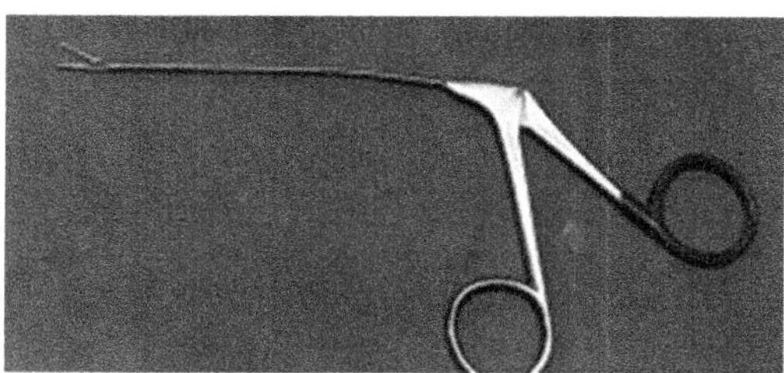

Fig. 25. Alligator forceps. (*Adapted from* Pfenninger JL, Fowler GC. Pfenninger & Fowler's procedures for primary care. 3rd edition. Philadelphia: Elsevier; 2011. p. 483–88.)

Table 3
Contraindications to etonogestrel implant use

Contraindication Per Package Labeling	USMEC Category	WHO Category	Comment
Known or suspected pregnancy	N/A	N/A	—
Current or past history of thrombosis or thrombotic disorders	2	2 if history of deep vein thrombosis or pulmonary emobolism (DVT/PE) or if DVT/PE and established on anticoagulant therapy 3 if acute DVT/PE	—
Undiagnosed abnormal genital bleeding	3	3	Category may be adjusted after evaluation
Known or suspected breast cancer, personal history of breast cancer, or other progestin-sensitive breast cancer, now or in the past	2 if undiagnosed mass 3 if past cancer and no evidence of current disease for 5 y 4 if current cancer	2 if undiagnosed mass 3 if past cancer and no evidence of current disease for 5 y 4 if current cancer	Evaluation for undiagnosed mass should be pursued as early as possible
Allergic reaction to any of the components of etonogestrel implant	N/A	N/A	—

discontinuation of the contraceptive implant; therefore thorough counseling on expected changes is of paramount importance. Once a patient has decided on a contraceptive implant, specific risks of insertion, including bleeding, infection, and pain or bruising at insertion site should be reviewed.

TECHNIQUE/PROCEDURE

Manufacture of the nonradiopaque etonogestrel implant (Implanon) was discontinued in 2011 with the introduction of the radiopaque etonogestrel implant (Nexplanon), making it the only implant available for insertion in the United States. This implant features a next-generation applicator (NGA) redesigned for correct, subdermal placement using 1 hand. All clinicians who insert and remove the etonogestrel implant must undergo training sponsored by the manufacturer before using the device in patients. This training includes an instructional video and supervised performance of 2 simulated insertions and removals in an artificial arm.

Insertion

The NGA (**Fig. 26**) has led to high clinician satisfaction with the functionality (91%–100%), design and technical aspects (96%–100%), and safety (96%–100%) of the insertion device. Insertion is very quick, with mean insertion time (plus or minus standard deviation) of 27.9 (29.3) seconds.[42]

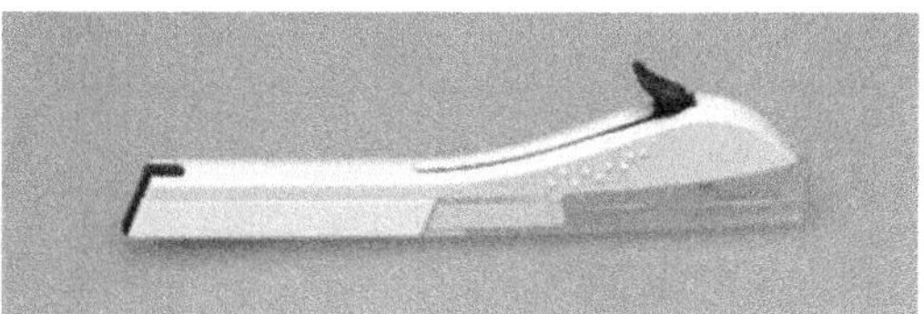

Fig. 26. Next-generation applicator. (*Courtesy of* Merck & Co., Inc.)

To begin, the patient is positioned supine on the examination table with the nondominant hand above the head, flexed at the elbow. The insertion site should be identified: 8 to 10 cm proximal to the medial epicondyle of the humerus on the inner site of the nondominant arm. This site is marked with either a pen or marker or with pressure from the tip of a retracted pen or needle cap. Insertion of the implant through a pen or marker site may lead to inadvertent tattooing of the patient. A second, guiding mark can be made several centimeters proximal to the insertion site as a guide during insertion (**Fig. 27**).

The insertion site is cleaned with antiseptic solution. The entire area of the expected insertion tunnel should be cleaned. Next, the insertion area is anesthetized; 2 to 3 cc of plain 1% lidocaine along the entire planned insertion tunnel should be sufficient. The implant is removed from the sterile packaging, and the transparent protective cap removed by sliding horizontally away from the needed. Care should be taken not to touch the purple slider until the needle is fully inserted to avoid premature release of the implant (**Fig. 28**).

With the free hand, the skin around the insertion site is stretched. The skin is punctured with the tip of the needle angled about 30° (**Fig. 29**). Improper angling of the inserter (>30°) may lead to deep insertions. The applicator is then lowered to a horizontal position. The skin should be tented with the needle and the needle slid to its full length. It is common for slight resistance to be felt, and this may increase when the needle is about half inserted. Excessive force should not be used, but one must be sure that the needle has been inserted to its full length. Failure to completely insert

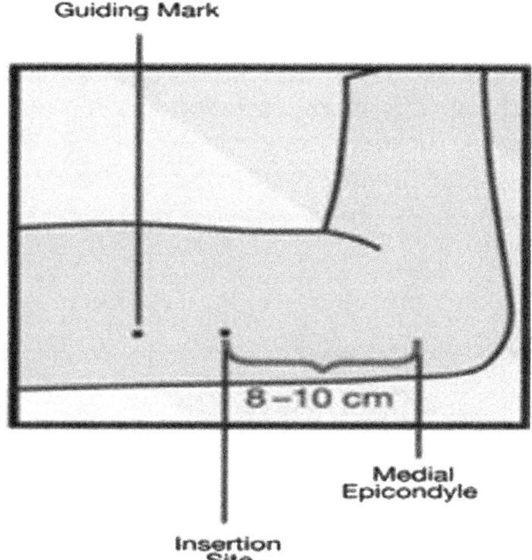

Fig. 27. A second, guiding mark should be made several centimeters proximal to the insertion site as a guide during insertion. (*Courtesy of* Merck & Co., Inc.)

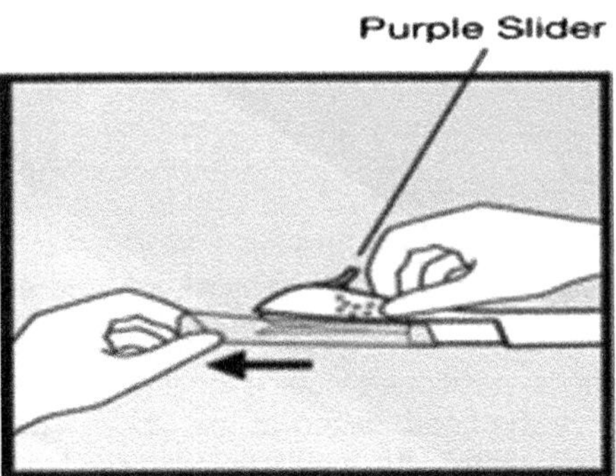

Fig. 28. One should remove the implant from the sterile packaging and remove the transparent protective cap by sliding horizontally away from the needed. Care should be taken not to touch the purple slider until the needle is fully inserted to avoid premature release of the implant. (*Courtesy of* Merck & Co., Inc.)

the needle will lead to incorrect implant placement and increased risk of expulsion (**Fig. 30**).[42]

With the needle inserted to its full length, the purple slider is unlocked by pushing slightly down, and moved fully back until it stops (**Fig. 31**). The applicator is then removed. The needle will be retracted and locked in the body of the applicator. The presence of the implant should be verified by palpation (**Fig. 32**).

The wound should be dressed with a small adhesive bandage over the insertion site and a pressure bandage for 24 to 48 hours to minimize bruising. A routine follow-up visit is not needed.

Removal

Removal of both etonogestrel implants is identical. Before attempting to remove an implant, the location must be identified. This is most often accomplished with palpation, but if nonpalpable, the implant should be localized. The manufacturer strongly discourages exploratory surgery without knowledge of the exact location of the implant.[38] Average removal time is about 3.5 minutes, with a range of 0.2 to 60 minutes in 1 study.[43]

To remove an implant, it must first be located by palpation, and the distal end marked. The site is cleaned with aseptic solution and the arm anesthetized where the incision will be made. To keep the implant closer to the skin surface, local

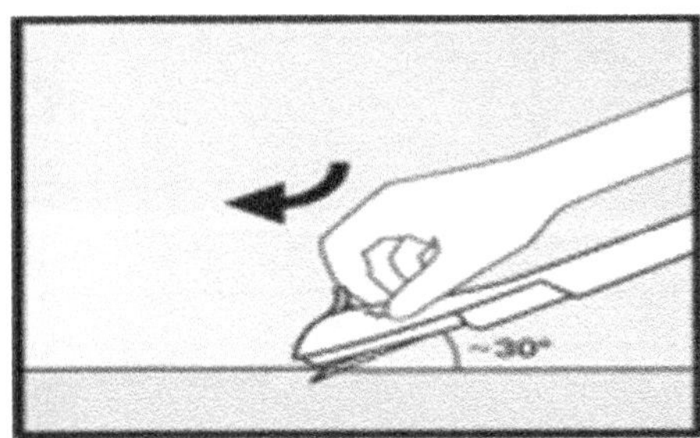

Fig. 29. With the free hand, the skin around the insertion site should be stretched. The skin should then be punctured with the tip of the needle angled about 30°. (*Courtesy of* Merck & Co., Inc.)

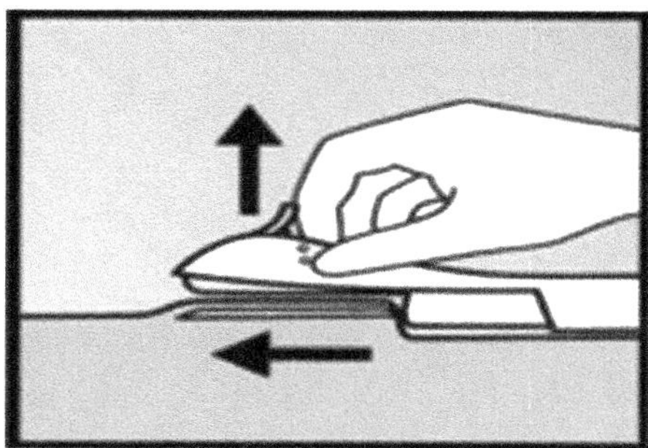

Fig. 30. The applicator should be lowered to a horizontal position. The skin should be tented with the needle and the needle slid to its full length. It is common for slight resistance to be felt, and this may increase when the needle is about half inserted. (*Courtesy of* Merck & Co., Inc.)

anesthetic (0.5 cc of 1% lidocaine) should be injected under the implant. If another implant is to be placed immediately, the entire track should be anesthetized.

The proximal end of the implant is pushed to raise the distal end closer to the skin surface. One should make a small (2–3 mm), longitudinal (parallel to the long axis of the implant) incision toward the elbow (**Fig. 33**). An 11-blade works well for this incision, and the incision can be extended if needed.

The implant is pushed toward the incision until the tip is visible. The implant is then grasped with forceps to remove (**Fig. 34**). Occasionally, a fibrous sheath will form around the implant. Should this occur, one should make an incision into the sheath before removing the implant (**Fig. 35**).

If the tip of the implant is not visible, one can insert the forceps into the incision, then flip to the other hand. A second set of forceps is then used to dissect the tissue around the implant and remove it (**Fig. 36**).

One should confirm that the entire implant has been removed (4 cm in length). The incision can be closed with a steri-strip. The wound should be dressed with a small adhesive bandage and a pressure bandage.

If desired, a new device can be placed immediately in the same insertion site. A routine follow-up visit is not needed.

Although the single-rod etonogestrel implant is the only implant available in the United States, clinicians may encounter patients from other parts of the world with implants. The LNG implant system (Norplant) is a set of 6 rods that was last available in the United States in 2002, but is still used in China (Sinoplant I).[41] Another LNG system

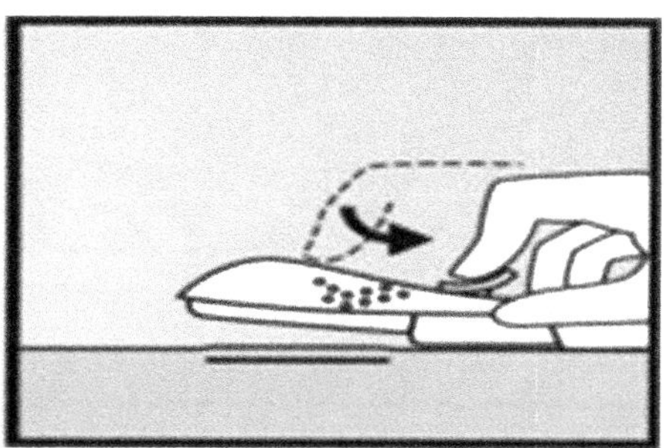

Fig. 31. With the needle inserted to its full length, the purple slider should be unlocked by pushing slightly down, and moving it fully back until it stops. (*Courtesy of* Merck & Co., Inc.)

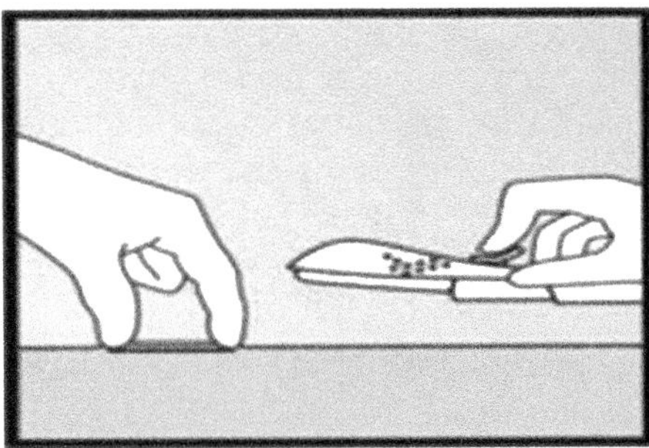

Fig. 32. The presence of the implant should be verified by palpation. (*Courtesy of* Merck & Co., Inc.)

(Sino-implant II) contains 2 rods and is available in Asia and Africa.[44] Clinicians should take a careful history of women who have had implants placed outside of the United States to determine which system was used and ensure complete removal of all implants.

COMPLICATIONS AND MANAGEMENT

Insertion

Nonpalpable implant

Incorrect placement of the etonogestrel implant can lead to deep insertions and nonpalpable implants. If the implant is nonpalpable, the patient should be advised to use back-up contraception until localization occurs. Partial expulsions have been reported immediately after insertion, always when the needle was not inserted to its full length.[42]

Nonradiopaque etonogestrel implants (Implanon) cannot be localized with 2-dimensional radiograph or computed tomography (CT) scan. First-line localization should be attempted with a high-frequency linear array transducer (10 MHz or greater).[45] These are not the typical transducers used in obstetrics and gynecology practices, but are routinely used for breast and musculoskeletal ultrasound. The appearance of the implant itself is not seen, rather a posterior acoustic shadow cast by the implant (**Fig. 37**).[46]

If ultrasound fails to locate a deeply inserted implant, magnetic resonance imaging (MRI) can be used. The implant will appear as a hypodense area/signal-void black spot (**Fig. 38**).[45]

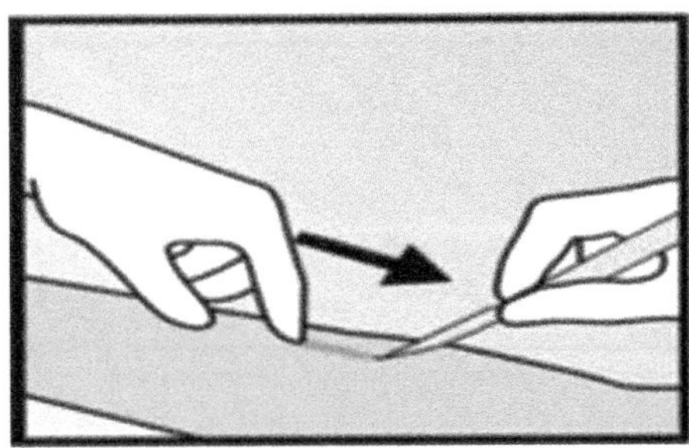

Fig. 33. One should push on the proximal end of the implant to raise the distal end closer to the skin surface. A small (2–3 mm), longitudinal (parallel to the long axis of the implant) incision should then be made toward the elbow. (*Courtesy of* Merck & Co., Inc.)

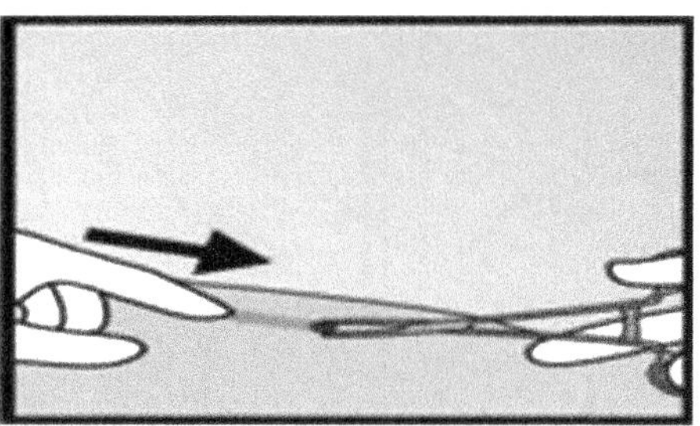

Fig. 34. One should push the implant toward the incision until the tip is visible. The implant then should be grasped with forceps to remove. (*Courtesy of* Merck & Co., Inc.)

Radiopaque etonogestrel implants (Nexplanon) are most easily identified on 2-dimensional radiograph imaging of the arm (**Fig. 39**). Two clinical trials studied a total of 114 women undergoing radiograph localization of the radiopaque implant before insertion and again before removal.[39,40] one hundred twelve (98%) were visible after insertion, and all were visible before removal. The nonvisualized implants after insertion were likely due to positioning of the arm at time of radiograph.

If imaging techniques fail to localize the implant, a serum etonogestrel level can be obtained by calling the manufacturer (Merck & Co., 1-877-467–5266).

Pain/paresthesia

Pain is the most common insertion complication reported in studies, with an incidence of 0.7% to 4.0%.[40,42,43,47–50] Adequate preinsertion anesthesia, as well as oral analgesics after the procedure can be used to minimize patient discomfort.

Improper placement has also been reported to result in neuropathy/paresthesia.[51] This emphasizes the importance of correct technique to ensure subdermal placement.

Implant site reactions (pain, swelling, redness, hematoma)

Implant site reactions are uncommon and typically resolve spontaneously. A study of 1716 women receiving the non-radiopaque etonogestrel implant showed 97.8% of women to have no abnormalities reported on the day of insertion.[48] The most common abnormality was pain in 1.9% of women, with <1% of women reporting swelling, redness or hematoma formation. A study of 301 women receiving the radiopaque implant had slightly higher numbers of abnormalities, with 91.4% reporting no reactions, 0.7% reporting pain, 1.3% reporting swelling, 4.0% reporting redness, and 3.3% reporting hematoma.[42]

Infection

Infection at implant site is a theoretical concern, but no large trials have reported cellulitis or insertion site infections as recorded complications.[42,43,47,48]

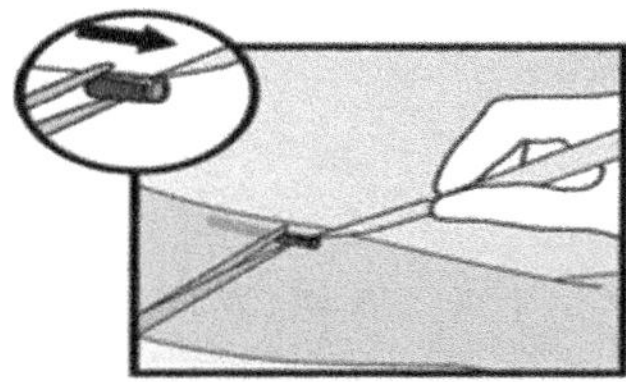

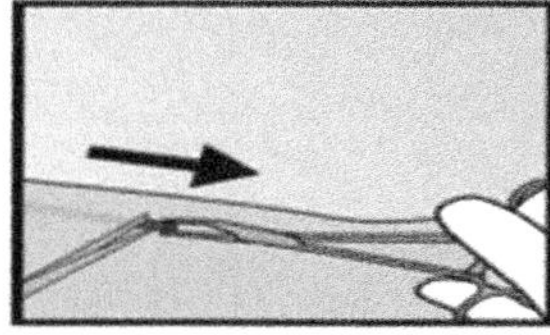

Fig. 35. Occasional, a fibrous sheath will form around the implant. Should this occur, an incision into the sheath should be made before removing the implant. (*Courtesy of* Merck & Co., Inc.)

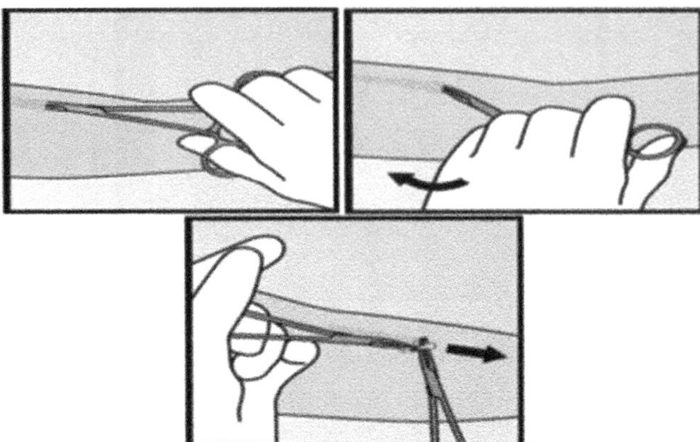

Fig. 36. If the tip of the implant is not visible, the forceps should be inserted into the incision. Then one should flip to the other hand. A second set of forceps is then used to dissect the tissue around the implant and remove it. (*Courtesy of* Merck & Co., Inc.)

Removal

Removal difficulties are uncommon, with reported incidences of 1.3% to 5.4%.[40,43,47,48] Complications include nonpalpable/deeply inserted implants, breakage of the implant during removal, and most commonly, presence of fibrotic tissue around the implant.

Removal should not be attempted if the implant is nonpalpable until localization has determined the exact location of the implant.[38,45] Nerve injuries have been reported from attempted office exploratory procedures to find nonpalpable implants.[52] Coordination with radiology or referral to a site with experience in image-guided removal may allow for office removal of radiologically localized implants. Otherwise, consideration should be given to referral to a surgeon familiar with the anatomy of the arm for removal.

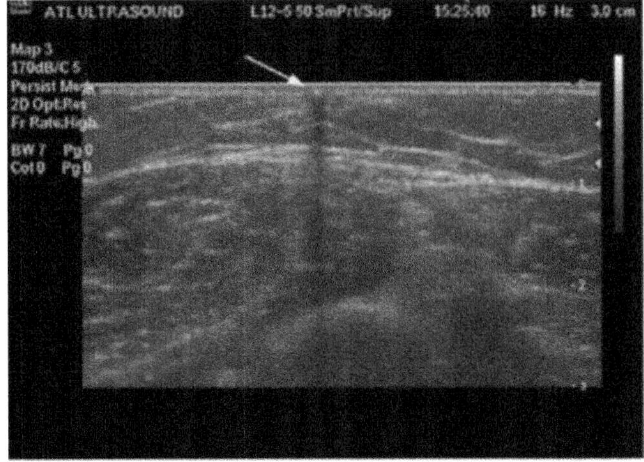

Fig. 37. The appearance of the implant itself is not seen, rather a posterior acoustic shadow cast by the implant.

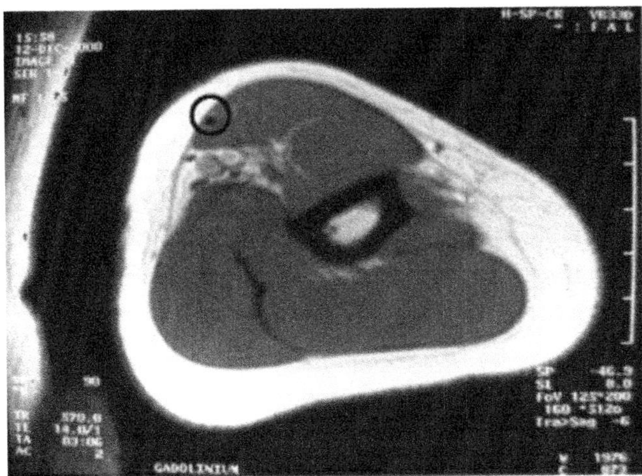

Fig. 38. If ultrasound fails to locate a deeply inserted implant, MRI can be used. The implant will appear as a hypodense area/signal-void black spot.

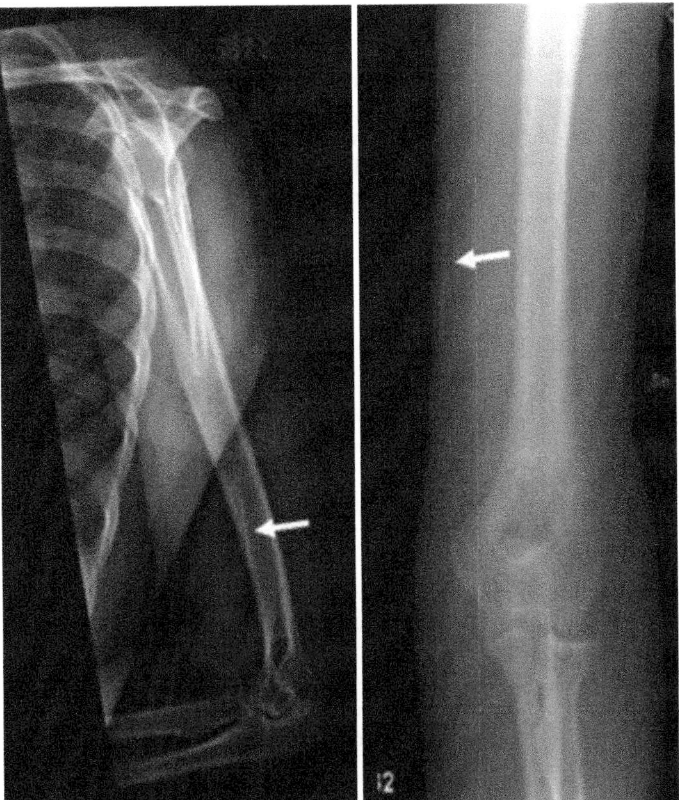

Fig. 39. Radiopaque etonogestrel implants (Nexplanon) are most easily identified on 2-dimensional radiograph imaging of the arm.

Table 4
Adverse reactions leading to discontinuation of treatment of etonogestrel implant

Adverse Reaction	All Studies (N = 942) (%)
Bleeding irregularities	11.1
Emotional lability	2.3
Weight increase	2.3
Headache	1.6
Acne	1.3
Depression	1.0

Data From Merck. Nexplanon (etonogestrel implant) prescribing information. 2011 [cited 2013 March 10]. Available at: http://www.merck.com/product/usa/pi_circulars/n/nexplanon/nexplanon_pi.pdf.

Outcomes

The etonogestrel implant is an exceedingly effective contraceptive. An integrated analysis of 11 studies with 942 women representing more than 1700 women–years of exposure found no pregnancies with the implant in situ.[47] Similarly, a more recent study of the radiopaque implant with 301 women representing 655 women–years of exposure found no pregnancies with the implant in situ.[40]

Changes in menstrual pattern are common, and the most frequently cited adverse reaction leading to removal (11.1%–14.8%).[38,47,53,54] The most common change in bleeding pattern is infrequent bleeding or spotting (33.6%–34.6%), followed by amenorrhea (22.2%–29.5%), prolonged bleeding or spotting (11.3%–17.7%), and frequent bleeding or spotting (3.9%–6.7%).[47,53] Counseling is therefore key in assuring that patients accept the risk of changes in menstrual pattern prior to insertion.[55] There is no evidence for a single best treatment regimen for menstrual changes while using the etonogestrel implants. Possible treatment strategies include a course of combined oral contraceptives, NSAIDs, high-dose cyclic progestin, or tranexamic acid.[56]

The most common adverse reactions leading to discontinuation are listed in **Table 4**.

SUMMARY

LARCs, such as IUDs and implants, are among the most effective forms of contraception available. There are few contraindications to their use, and insertion and removal are straightforward procedures that are well tolerated in the outpatient office setting.

The American College of Obstetrician and Gynecologists recognizes high upfront patient costs as a barrier to LARC use and advocates for coverage of all contraceptive methods by all insurance plans.[57] In July 2011, the Institute of Medicine published an expert committee report on preventative services for women that should be considered in developing comprehensive health guidelines.[58] It defined preventative services as "measures—including medications, procedures, devices, tests, education, and counseling—shown to improve well-being and/or decrease the likelihood or delay the onset of a targeted disease or condition." Among these services are the full range of FDA-approved contraceptive devices. The following month, the Department of Health and Human Services incorporated these recommendations into preventative services covered by health plans under the Patient Protection and Affordable Care Act (ACA), without cost sharing by the patient.[59] While there are continuing legal battles over the ACA, it is hoped that with its full implementation over the coming years women will have increased access to these safe, effective forms of birth control.

REFERENCES

1. Finer LB, Zolna MR. Unintended pregnancy in the United States: incidence and disparities, 2006. Contraception 2011;84(5):478–85.
2. Singh S, Sedgh G, Hussain R. Unintended pregnancy: worldwide levels, trends, and outcomes. Stud Fam Plann 2010;41(4):241–50.
3. Healthypeople.Gov. Healthy people 2020, family planning objectives. Available at: http://healthypeople.gov/2020/topicsobjectives2020/objectiveslist.aspx?topicId=13. Accessed April 1, 2013.
4. Finer LB, Jerman J, Kavanaugh ML. Changes in use of long-acting contraceptive methods in the United States, 2007–2009. Fertil Steril 2012;984:893–7.
5. Trussell J. Contraceptive failure in the United States. Contraception 2011;835: 397–404.
6. Bayer Healthcare Pharmaceuticals Inc. Skyla prescribing information. 2013. Available at: http://labeling.bayerhealthcare.com/html/products/pi/Skyla_PI.pdf. Accessed April 1, 2013.
7. Bayer Healthcare Pharmaceuticals Inc. Mirena prescribing information. Available at: http://labeling.bayerhealthcare.com/html/products/pi/Mirena_PI.pdf. Accessed April 1, 2013.
8. Seeber B, Ziehr SC, Gschließer A, et al. Quantitative levonorgestrel plasma level measurements in patients with regular and prolonged use of the levonorgestrel-releasing intrauterine system. Contraception 2012;864:345–9.
9. Hidalgo MM, Hidalgo-Regina C, Bahamondes MV, et al. Serum levonorgestrel levels and endometrial thickness during extended use of the levonorgestrel-releasing intrauterine system. Contraception 2009;801:84–9.
10. Sivin I, Stern J, Coutinho E, et al. Prolonged intrauterine contraception: a seven-year randomized study of the levonorgestrel 20 mcg/day (lng 20) and the copper T380 Ag IUDS. Contraception 1991;445:473–80.
11. Sivin I. Utility and drawbacks of continuous use of a copper T IUD for 20 years. Contraception 2007;75(Suppl 6):S70–5.
12. United Nations Development Programme, United Nations Population Fund, World Health Organization, et al. Long-term reversible contraception: twelve years of experience with the TCu380A and TCu220C. Contraception 1997; 56(6):341–52.
13. Wu S, Godfrey EM, Wojdyla D, et al. Copper T380A intrauterine device for emergency contraception: a prospective, multicentre, cohort clinical trial. BJOG 2010;117(10):1205–10.
14. Ewies AA, Alfhaily F. Use of levonorgestrel-releasing intrauterine system in the prevention and treatment of endometrial hyperplasia. Obstet Gynecol Surv 2012;67(11):726–33.
15. Centers for Disease Control and Prevention CDC. U.S. Medical eligibility criteria for contraceptive use, 2010. MMWR Recomm Rep 2010;59(RR–4):1–85.
16. World Health Organization. Medical eligibility criteria for contraceptive use. 2009. 4th. Available at: http://www.who.int/reproductivehealth/publications/family_planning/9789241563888/en/index.htm. Accessed March 10, 2013.
17. Whiteman MK, Tyler CP, Folger SG, et al. When can a woman have an intrauterine device inserted? A systematic review. Contraception 2013;87(5):666–73.
18. O'Hanley K, Huber DH. Postpartum IUDs: keys for success. Contraception 1992;45(4):351–61.
19. Speroff L, Mishell DR. The postpartum visit: it's time for a change in order to optimally initiate contraception. Contraception 2008;78(2):90–8.

20. Kapp N, Curtis KM. Intrauterine device insertion during the postpartum period: a systematic review. Contraception 2009;80(4):327–36.
21. Osborn NG, Wright RC. Effect of preoperative scrub on the bacterial flora of the endocervix and vagina. Obstet Gynecol 1977;50(2):148–51.
22. Mody SK, Kiley J, Rademaker A, et al. Pain control for intrauterine device insertion: a randomized trial of 1% lidocaine paracervical block. Contraception 2012;86(6):704–9.
23. Allen RH, Bartz D, Grimes DA, et al. Interventions for pain with intrauterine device insertion. Cochrane Database Syst Rev 2009;(3):CD007373.
24. Maguire K, Davis A, Rosario Tejeda L, et al. Intracervical lidocaine gel for intrauterine device insertion: a randomized controlled trial. Contraception 2012;86(3):214–9.
25. Nelson AL, Fong JK. Intrauterine infusion of lidocaine does not reduce pain scores during IUD insertion. Contraception 2013;88(1):37–40.
26. McNicholas CP, Madden T, Zhao Q, et al. Cervical lidocaine for IUD insertional pain: a randomized controlled trial. Am J Obstet Gynecol 2012;207(5):384.e1–6.
27. Kaislasuo J, Suhonen S, Gissler M, et al. Intrauterine contraception: incidence and factors associated with uterine perforation—a population-based study. Hum Reprod 2012;279:2658–63.
28. Adoni A, Ben Chetrit A. The management of intrauterine devices following uterine perforation. Contraception 1991;43(1):77–81.
29. Markovitch O, Klein Z, Gidoni Y, et al. Extrauterine mislocated IUD: is surgical removal mandatory? Contraception 2002;66(2):105–8.
30. Kaislasuo J, Suhonen S, Gissler M, et al. Uterine perforation caused by intrauterine devices: clinical course and treatment. Hum Reprod 2013;28(6):1546–51.
31. Dean G, Schwarz EB. Intrauterine contraceptives (IUCs). In: Hatcher RA, Trussell J, Nelson A, et al, editors. Contraceptive technology. Atlanta (GA): Ardent Media, Inc; 2011. p. 147–92.
32. Zhang J, Feldblum PJ, Chi IC, et al. Risk factors for copper T IUD expulsion: an epidemiologic analysis. Contraception 1992;46(5):427–33.
33. Brahmi D, Steenland MW, Renner RM, et al. Pregnancy outcomes with an IUD in situ: a systematic review. Contraception 2012;85(2):131–9.
34. Farley TM, Rowe PJ, Meirik O, et al. Intrauterine devices and pelvic inflammatory disease: an international perspective. Lancet 1992;339(8796):785–8.
35. Workowski KA, Berman S, Centers for Disease Control and Prevention. Sexually transmitted diseases treatment guidelines, 2010. MMWR Recomm Rep 2010;59(RR–12):63–7.
36. Grimes DA, Lopez LM, Schulz KF. Antibiotic prophylaxis for intrauterine contraceptive device insertion. Cochrane Database Syst Rev 2001;(2):CD001327.
37. Westhoff C. IUDs and colonization or infection with actinomyces. Contraception 2007;75(Suppl 6):S48–50.
38. Merck. Nexplanon (etonogestrel implant) prescribing information. 2011. Available at: http://www.merck.com/product/usa/pi_circulars/n/nexplanon/nexplanon_pi.pdf. Accessed March 10, 2013.
39. Schnabel P, Merki-Feld GS, Malvy A, et al. Bioequivalence and x-ray visibility of a radiopaque etonogestrel implant versus a non-radiopaque implant. Clin Drug Investig 2012;32(6):413–22.
40. Mommers E, Blum GF, Gent TG, et al. Nexplanon, a radiopaque etonogestrel implant in combination with a next-generation applicator: 3-year results of a noncomparative multicenter trial. Am J Obstet Gynecol 2012;207(5):388.e1–6.

41. Raymond E. Contraceptive implants. In: Hatcher RA, Trussell J, Nelson A, et al, editors. Contraceptive technology. Atlanta (GA): Ardent Media Inc; 2011. p. 193–207.
42. Mansour D, Mommers E, Teede H, et al. Clinician satisfaction and insertion characteristics of a new applicator to insert radiopaque Implanon: an open-label, noncontrolled, multicenter trial. Contraception 2010;82(3):243–9.
43. Levine JP, Sinofsky FE, Christ MF. Assessment of implanon insertion and removal. Contraception 2008;78(5):409–17.
44. Steiner MJ, Lopez LM, Grimes DA, et al. Sino-implant (II)—a levonorgestrel-releasing two-rod implant: systematic review of the randomized controlled trials. Contraception 2010;81(3):197–201.
45. Shulman LP, Gabriel H. Management and localization strategies for the nonpalpable implanon rod. Contraception 2006;73(4):325–30.
46. Lantz A, Nosher JL, Pasquale S, et al. Ultrasound characteristics of subdermally implanted Implanon contraceptive rods. Contraception 1997;56(5):323–7.
47. Darney P, Patel A, Rosen K, et al. Safety and efficacy of a single-rod etonogestrel implant (Implanon): results from 11 international clinical trials. Fertil Steril 2009;91(5):1646–53.
48. Mascarenhas L. Insertion and removal of implanon. Contraception 1998; 58(Suppl 6):79S–83S.
49. Urbancsek J. An integrated analysis of nonmenstrual adverse events with Implanon. Contraception 1998;58(Suppl 6):109S–15S.
50. Croxatto HB, Urbancsek J, Massai R, et al. A multicentre efficacy and safety study of the single contraceptive implant Implanon. Hum Reprod 1999;14(4):976–81.
51. Brown M, Britton J. Neuropathy associated with etonogestrel implant insertion. Contraception 2012;86(5):591–3.
52. Gillies R, Scougall P, Nicklin S. Etonogestrel implants: case studies of median nerve injury following removal. Aust Fam Physician 2011;40(10):799–800.
53. Mansour D, Korver T, Marintcheva-Petrova M, et al. The effects of Implanon on menstrual bleeding patterns. Eur J Contracept Reprod Health Care 2008;13: 13–28.
54. Casey PM, Long ME, Marnach ML, et al. Bleeding related to etonogestrel subdermal implant in a US population. Contraception 2011;83(5):426–30.
55. Halpern V, Lopez LM, Grimes DA, et al. Strategies to improve adherence and acceptability of hormonal methods of contraception. Cochrane Database Syst Rev 2011;(4):CD004317.
56. Mansour D, Bahamondes L, Critchley H, et al. The management of unacceptable bleeding patterns in etonogestrel-releasing contraceptive implant users. Contraception 2011;83(3):202–10.
57. American College of Obstetricians and Gynecologists Committee on Gynecologic Practice, Long-Acting Reversible Contraception Working Group. ACOG committee opinion no. 450: increasing use of contraceptive implants and intrauterine devices to reduce unintended pregnancy. Obstet Gynecol 2009;114(6): 1434–8.
58. Institute of Medicine. Clinical preventative services for women: Closing the gaps. July 2011. Available at: http://www.iom.edu/~/media/Files/Report%20Files/2011/Clinical-Preventive-Services-for-Women-Closing-the-Gaps/preventiveservicesforwomenreportbrief_updated2.pdf. Accessed March 22, 2013.
59. Health Resources and Services Administration. Women's preventative services: required health plan coverage guidelines. Available at: http://www.hrsa.gov/womensguidelines. Accessed March 22, 2013.

Performance of a Colposcopic Examination, a Loop Electrosurgical Procedure, and Cryotherapy of the Cervix

John G. Pierce Jr, MD*, Saweda Bright, MD

KEYWORDS

• Colposcopy • Loop electrosurgical • Cervical cryotherapy

KEY POINTS

- The colposcope is a magnifying instrument used to examine the uterine cervix, lower genital tract, and anogenital area.
- Since the 1960's colposcopy has become the accepted method of evaluation for abnormal PAP smears and other abnormalities of the cervix.
- The goal of colposcopy is to direct biopsies to the most abnormal appearing area(s), or if no abnormalities are seen, to randomly sample the transformation zone to rule out dysplasia.
- The results from the Pap test, the colposcopic impression, and the histologic evaluation of the biopsies will provide the final diagnosis to determine appropriate management.
- Loop electrocautery and cervical cryotherapy are the most common methods utilized to treat cervical dysplasia.

The colposcope is a magnifying instrument used to examine the uterine cervix, lower genital tract, and anogenital area. Colposcopy was first introduced in the United States by Emmer with a publication in 1931.[1] It was not until the 1960s with improved understanding of carcinogenesis that colposcopy gained more acceptance. Since that time, colposcopy has had great success as a diagnostic test for the abnormal Pap test to determine the location and extent of cervical intraepithelial lesions (CIN).[2]

The goal of colposcopy is to direct biopsies to the most abnormal appearing area(s), or if no abnormalities are seen, to randomly sample the transformation zone (TZ) to rule out dysplasia. The results from the Pap test, the colposcopic impression, and the histologic evaluation of the biopsies will provide the final diagnosis to determine

Department of Obstetrics and Gynecology, Virginia Commonwealth University Health System, 1250 East Marshall Street, PO Box 980034, Richmond, VA 23298-0034, USA
* Corresponding author.
E-mail address: jpierce2@mcvh-vcu.edu

Obstet Gynecol Clin N Am 40 (2013) 731–757
http://dx.doi.org/10.1016/j.ogc.2013.08.008
0889-8545/13/$ – see front matter Published by Elsevier Inc.

appropriate management. This article reviews the colposcopic examination for practitioners.

PREPARATION

In preparation for the colposcopic examination, it is imperative to have a prepared examining room with a fully functioning colposcope and all of the necessary supplies and equipment. Two major types of colposcopes exist: the traditional optical colposcope and the newer video colposcope.

The optical colposcope may be a single-objective versus double-objective lens (**Fig. 1**). Although a single-lens colposcope is adequate, the double-objective lens is preferred by most colposcopists, providing true stereoscopic images. The video colposcope uses a monitor to enable the colposcopist and often the patient to view the cervix on a video screen rather than through the eyepiece (**Fig. 2**).

The instruments and supplies must be well organized and readily available with an experienced assistant to help. Supplies that are needed include metal or disposable vaginal specula of various sizes, lateral sidewall retractors, 3% to 5% acetic acid, Lugol iodine, cotton tip applicators and large cotton swabs, endocervical specula of varying sizes, biopsy forceps (Kevorkian or Tischler or baby Tischler) (**Fig. 3**), endocervical brushes and/or curettes, tissue forceps, biopsy specimen containers with fixative, hemostatic agents (silver nitrate sticks, ferric subsulfate [Monsel] solution/paste), and latex/latex-free gloves (**Box 1**).

The most common indication for a colposcopy is an abnormal Pap test. The indications for colposcopy are well documented, with the most recent guidelines for management of the abnormal cervical cancer screening tests presented by the American Society for Colposcopy and Cervical Pathology (ASCCP) in 2012.[3] Some

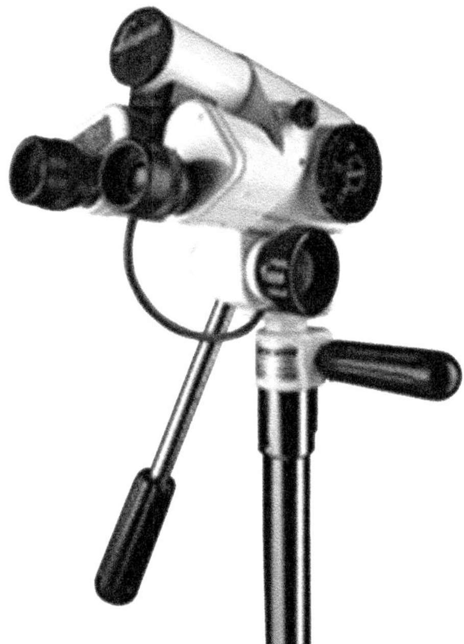

Fig. 1. Optical colposcope with a double objective lens. (*Courtesy of* Welch Allyn Inc., Skaneateles Falls, NY; with permission.)

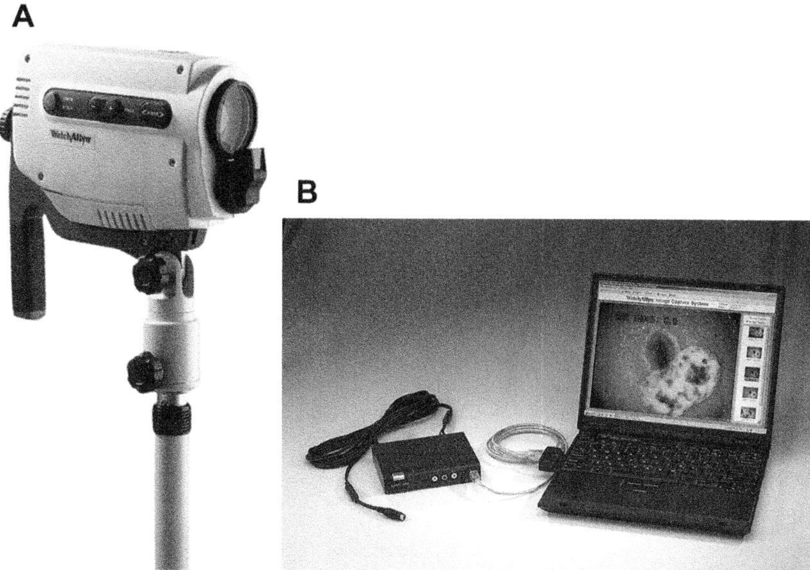

Fig. 2. Video colposcope (*A*) with a laptop monitor (*B*). (*Courtesy of* Welch Allyn Inc., Skaneateles Falls, NY; with permission.)

of the most common cervical cancer screening results requiring colposcopy for further evaluation include unsatisfactory cytology with positive high-risk human papilloma virus (+HR HPV) in women older than 30 years, ASC-US (atypical squamous cells of undetermined significance) with +HR HPV, persistent atypical squamous cells (ASCs), and low-grade squamous intraepithelial lesion (LGSIL). ASCs cannot exclude high-grade squamous intraepithelial lesion (ASC-H), high-grade intraepithelial lesion (HSIL), and atypical glandular cells (AGC).

Other indications for colposcopy include a gross or palpable cervical mass or ulcer, clinical suspicion for cervical cancer on visual inspection, history of in utero

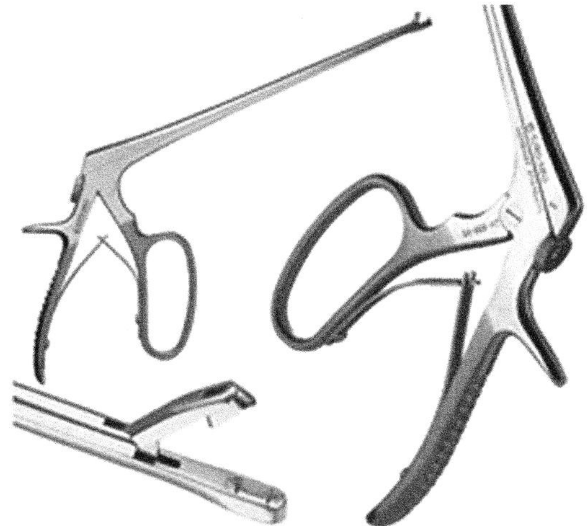

Fig. 3. Biopsy forceps. (Product images provided courtesy of Cooper Surgical, Inc.)

Box 1
Colposcopy equipment, materials, and supplies

- Colposcope: standard single or binocular optical lens or video colposcope, 300-mm focal length, variable magnification, red-free filter
- Metal or disposable vaginal specula of various sizes:
  - Short and long Pederson specula
  - Short and long Graves specula
  - Cusco or Collin speculum
  - Coated, electrically resistant specula containing tubing to evacuate smoke are best for LEEP
- Lateral sidewall retractors (if needed)
- 3%–5% acetic acid
- Lugol iodine
- Cotton tip applicators and large cotton swabs
- Endocervical specula of varying sizes (if needed)
- Biopsy forceps (multiple types including Kevorkian or Tischler or baby Tischler)
- Endocervical brushes and/or curettes
- Tissue forces
- Biopsy specimen containers with fixative
- Hemostatic agents: silver nitrate sticks, ferric subsulfate (Monsel) solution or paste
- Latex and latex-free gloves for patients who have a latex allergy

diethylstilbesterol (DES) exposure, unexplained lower genital tract bleeding, patient concern over partner with lower genital tract neoplasia or condyloma, vulvar or vaginal HPV-associated lesions, and postsurgical follow-up examination.[4]

There are no clear contraindications to a colposcopic examination. Colposcopy and biopsy are safe for immunosuppressed patients and for women taking anticoagulant medications. The only clear contraindications during colposcopy is an endocervical sampling in pregnant women, as that may introduce infection or cause rupture of the membranes. Women with acute cervicitis or severe vaginitis are usually evaluated with wet prep and cervical testing for infection, then treated before colposcopy to improve accuracy. In addition, it is easier to do a colposcopy when a patient is not having heavier menstrual flow. If there are concerns that the patient will not return for colposcopy after the infection is treated or after menstruation is finished, the colposcopy can still be performed.

When patients are notified of an abnormal Pap test, counseling and guidance are needed to ease the patient's anxiety and to facilitate a good, trusting relationship. Patients need to know what abnormality was found and how colposcopy is used to clarify the diagnosis and plan treatment. A brief explanation is important for the patient to know what to expect and how to prepare for the visit. Using an educational pamphlet is often an informative aid and a helpful visual picture for the patient to understand the procedure. This same pamphlet can be used in the office just before the procedure to review the colposcopy in greater detail and to obtain consent.

To prepare for the colposcopy, patients should preferably avoid intravaginal products, medications, douching, and sexual intercourse for 24 hours before the colposcopy.[4] Patients should be encouraged to have a spouse, friend, or relative accompany them for the examination.

Premedication before the colposcopy is not required. Although taking oral pain-relieving drugs (nonsteroidal anti-inflammatory drugs [NSAIDs]) before treatment on the cervix in the colposcopy clinic is recommended by most guidelines, evidence from some small trials in the Cochrane Review does not show that this practice reduces pain during the procedure.[5] The use of ibuprofen has been shown to be equivalent to placebo for pain control during the procedure.[6] Rarely, an anxiolytic medication may be used to treat for significant anxiety.

A brief history is recommended before the colposcopy, and the use of a standardized note will facilitate good documentation (Appendix A). Medical history should include major medical problems, such as diabetes, immunosuppression, human immunodeficiency virus (HIV) infection, hematologic or bleeding dyscrasias, tobacco use, and allergies. Helping the patient understand the association of smoking with cervical dysplasia and cancer facilitates an open discussion of risks of smoking and highlights the need for cessation. The gynecologic history should include the last menstrual period, menstrual history, postcoital bleeding, pregnancy history, age of sexual debut, number of lifetime sexual partners, history of in utero DES exposure, method of contraception, previous sexually transmitted infections (STIs) or pelvic inflammatory disease (PID), and current symptoms of vaginal discharge. Knowing the patient's history of previous HPV infections, abnormal Pap tests, and evaluations or treatments for dysplasia is advised.

As part of the consent process, the practitioner should begin with a full explanation of the procedure. Informed consent is usually done in writing but may also be obtained verbally followed by clear documentation. Research shows that patients' emotions can be negative and positive.[7] Negative feelings of fear, anxiety, and embarrassment are often described during the appointment or related to the outcome of the examination. Positive emotions such as relief, satisfaction, and relaxation were felt during the colposcopy when there is a positive attitude of the staff and good, empathetic care. An explanation of the procedure to the patient might be as follows:

> *The colposcopic exam is sort of a 'fancy Pap test.' A speculum is placed in the vagina similar to a Pap test. This 'telescope-like' device, a colposcope, is used to examine the vagina and cervix. A vinegar solution (acetic acid) is placed on the cervix with a cotton tip applicator, which may cause a mild burning sensation. This solution allows us to see the abnormal areas in order to take a biopsy. Most patients feel no or minimal pain with the biopsy. Some women may feel small to moderate pain with the biopsy but severe pain is very unusual.[6] Sometimes we need to take an additional biopsy of the inside of the cervix (the endocervical curettage), which might cause menstrual cramping or pain. Overall, the exam should take approximately 10 to 15 minutes. We will talk to you throughout the examination and I want to know how you are doing... Do you have any questions?*

COLPOSCOPIC TECHNIQUE

The approach to colposcopy should be systematic and orderly. The main purpose for the colposcopy is to identify invasive or preinvasive neoplastic lesions for colposcopically directed biopsy and subsequent management. To ensure a complete examination, several objectives must be fulfilled[4]:

- Visualize the cervix, vagina, vulva, and perianal area
- Identify the squamocolumnar junction (SCJ) and the TZ
- Determine whether the colposcopy is satisfactory or unsatisfactory

- Identify and assess size, shape, contour, location, and extent of the neoplastic lesion(s)
- Identify and sample the most severe lesions
- Sample the endocervical canal (unless the patient is pregnant)
- Correlate Pap test, biopsy report, and colposcopic impression
- Plan appropriate treatment plan
- Communicate findings to patient

The ASCCP and expert colposcopists have divided the examination into 4 distinct tasks[4]: (1) visualization of the cervix; (2) assessment of the cervix and abnormalities; (3) sampling with appropriate biopsies; and (4) correlation of cytologic, histologic, and colposcopic findings. This approach facilitates learning colposcopy and applying consistent colposcopic principles needed for a complete examination.

VISUALIZATION OF THE CERVIX

1. Selection and placement of the speculum
2. Complete visualization of the cervix
3. Focusing of the colposcope
4. Additional test collection if needed
5. Removing mucous or blood from cervix
6. Application of acetic acid or Lugol solution

With an established "doctor–patient relationship," the examiner maximizes trust and confidence. The patient should be as relaxed as possible in the dorsal lithotomy position with her feet in the foot rests ("stirrups"). Her buttocks must be at the edge of the bed, allowing room for the speculum after placement. The examining table should be adjusted so that the cervix will be at a comfortable height for the practitioner to view the lower genital tract through the colposcope. The widest speculum that can be well-tolerated by the patient provides the best exposure of the cervix. Once the speculum is placed into the vagina and the cervix is visualized, the blades of the speculum are opened as wide as possible without causing discomfort. Communication with the patient during the examination provides reassurance, sets expectations, and improves confidence in the practitioner performing the examination.

If good visualization is not achieved initially, the choice of speculum must be reassessed. A longer or wider speculum may be chosen to replace the first one. If the sidewalls of the vagina converge toward the center of the visual field, the colposcopist can use either a lateral sidewall retractor (**Fig. 4**) or place a condom or finger of a latex glove over the speculum. With the lateral sidewall retractor, the retractor is placed first to retract the sidewalls, then the speculum is inserted in the vagina and opened to visualize the cervix. In using the condom or finger of a latex glove, the "sleeve" is placed over the blades of the speculum, then the speculum is inserted and opened to visualize the cervix with lateral support from the condom or latex finger. These tricks are more commonly needed with the obese patient or with some degree of prolapse.

When significant vaginal discharge or cervical friability is present, additional specimens should now be obtained. Specimens may be sent for Gram stain, culture, wet mount, pH, whiff test, and/or screens for *Neisseria gonorrhea* and *Chlamydia trachomatis*. A repeat Pap test can be obtained, but will not usually provide additional information with the colposcopy.

Once the cervix is adequately visualized and specimens obtained, the examiner should change gloves so clean gloves are used to position the colposcope, minimizing contamination. Most colposcopes will have a focal length of the objective lens at

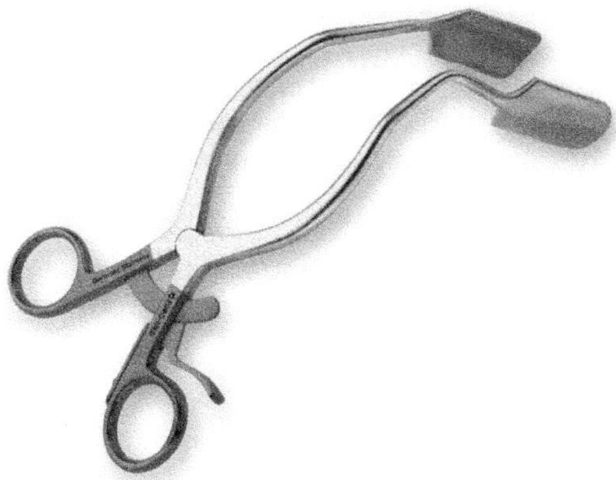

Fig. 4. Lateral sidewall retractor for vagina. (Product images provided courtesy of Cooper Surgical, Inc.)

300 mm so the distance between the lens and the cervix will be approximately 12 inches. Initially, the colposcope is adjusted on low-power magnification at 2 to 4 times. The focus can be achieved by moving the colposcope head closer or farther away from the cervix. Once the cervix is focused manually, higher magnification can be obtained by incremental increases in power magnification. The magnification can be sequentially increased to 6 to 15 times, then further adjusted with the fine-focus handle or moving the colposcope closer or farther away from the site in view.

The video colposcope is adjusted with a zoom control until maximum magnification is obtained; the fine focus is then adjusted in either direction. For the video colposcope, focus will usually be maintained throughout the entire magnification range once these steps have been completed, as long as the video colposcope or target is not moved.

Sometimes the focus of the entire cervix is difficult to view because of the angle of cervix relative to the colposcope. By placing a large moistened cotton tip swab in one of the vaginal fornices and applying pressure, the cervix can be manipulated, providing clearer visualization.

Some colposcopists will apply normal saline with a swab to moisten the cervix and remove mucous or discharge that is present. Examination with the saline allows for visualization of leukoplakia and abnormal blood vessels. Many colposcopists skip the assessment with normal saline and begin with applying 3% to 5% acetic acid to the cervix. This application is applied liberally with a large cotton swab that is soaked with the acetic acid. Two to 3 applications of acetic acid over a few minutes is often needed to allow the full effect on the epithelium to take place. The acetic acid is a mucolytic agent that is thought to exert its effect by reversibly clumping nuclear chromatin. This causes lesions to assume various shades of white depending on the degree of abnormal nuclear density. Therefore, gentle bathing of the cervix with the acetic acid swabs will improve colposcopic viewing.

The vagina and cervix should be evaluated on low magnification to look for acetowhite lesions. The cervix can be manipulated or moved around with a soaked swab so that the vagina and the fornices are fully examined. The cervix should be seen in its entirety before concentrating on the TZ. If lesions are recognized on low power, higher magnification at 10 to 15 times allows for closer examination.

Although optional and not used by all colposcopists, Lugol iodine solution is another contrast agent available. It is most beneficial when the acetic acid examination is inadequate or to stain the vagina, as vaginal lesions are more difficult to see than cervical lesions. Lugol solution stains mature squamous cells a dark brown color in estrogenized women, as the cells contain a high concentration of glycogen. Dysplastic cells have lower glycogen content, failing to fully stain and therefore appearing various shades of yellow. Normal columnar epithelium, immature squamous metaplastic epithelium, and neoplastic epithelium will not stain with Lugol solution. Columnar or immature squamous metaplastic epithelium will appear light yellow or reddish pink. Neoplastic epithelium has a range of staining, with CIN 1 being an orange to yellow color and higher grades of dysplasia staining a brighter yellow to white color.

ASSESSMENT OF THE CERVIX AND ABNORMALITIES

1. Classifying the colposcopy as adequate or inadequate
2. Identification of the SCJ and the TZ
3. Identification of epithelial abnormalities
4. Determining the size, shape, contour, location, and extent of the lesions

Using consistent terminology for a colposcopic assessment is crucial for clinical care and research. Terms in this article follow the 2011 International Federation of Cervical Pathology and Colposcopy (**Table 1**).[8] The initial statement about every

Table 1
2011 International Federation of Cervical Pathology and Colposcopic Terminology of the cervix

	Pattern
General assessment	Adequate or inadequate for the reason… Squamocolumnar junction visibility: completely visible, partially visible, not visible Transformation zone types 1, 2, 3
Normal colposcopic findings	Original squamous epithelium: mature, atrophic Columnar epithelium; ectopy, ectropion Metaplastic squamous epithelium; Nabothian cysts; crypt (gland) openings Deciduosis in pregnancy
Abnormal colposcopic findings	Location of the lesion: • Inside or outside the transformation zone • Location of the lesion by clock position Size of the lesion: number of cervical quadrants the lesion covers Size of the lesion as percentage of cervix Grade 1 (minor): fine mosaic; fine punctation; thin acetowhite epithelium; irregular, geographic border Grade 2 (major): sharp border; inner border sign; ridge sign; dense acetowhite epithelium; coarse mosaic; coarse punctuation; rapid appearance of acetowhitening; cuffed crypt (gland) openings Nonspecific: leukoplakia (keratosis, hyperkeratosis), erosion Lugol staining (Schiller test): stained or nonstained
Suspicious for invasion	Atypical vessels Additional signs: fragile vessels, irregular surface, exophytic lesion, necrosis, ulceration (necrotic), tumor, or gross neoplasm
Miscellaneous findings	Congenital transformation zone, condyloma, polyp (ectocervical or endocervical), inflammation, stenosis, congenital anomaly, posttreatment consequence, endometriosis

Data from Bornstein J, Bentley J, Bosze P, et al. 2011 Colposcopic Terminology of the International Federation for Cervical Pathology and Colposcopy. Obstet Gynecol 2012;120(1):166–72.

colposcopic examination should be described as either "adequate" or "Inadequate for the reason…." An adequate colposcopy is one that visualizes the SCJ in 360° and the margins of any visible lesion. An "adequate colposcopy" implies a complete examination in which all areas were adequately assessed. An "inadequate colposcopy" communicates that not all of the areas were visualized and an additional excisional procedure may be necessary.

To begin assessing the cervix, clear understanding of the TZ is essential. The TZ is the area between the original SCJ and the current SCJ. The current SCJ should be identified in 360°. The original SCJ is further outside of the current SCJ and defined as the position of the SCJ on the ectocervix at birth. The original SCJ cannot be clearly known but may be surmised in young patients if squamous metaplasia is visible with gland openings or Nabothian cysts. Even if it cannot be clearly determined, looking closely at the TZ is critical, as this is the area most likely to contain cervical neoplasia. The area contains both mature and immature metaplastic epithelium. The immature metaplasia is more susceptible to cellular insult by infection with HPV. This insult can divert the normal maturation process, leading to neoplastic transformation.

If the current SCJ cannot be clearly visualized at the external os, 3 main options can be tried to improve visualization. First, adjustment of the speculum should be considered, as this may improve the exposure or the angle of the visualization. Second, moistened cotton swabs can move the cervix or push on the fornices to change the angle of the view down the cervical os. Also, smaller cotton tip applicators can push or open the external os, slightly improving visualization. The third option is to use an endocervical speculum (**Fig. 5**). The endocervical speculum is placed within the external os and opened slightly. It may then be rotated around to visualize the entire SCJ. Although the SCJ can frequently be visualized with one of these methods, adequate visualization of the SCJ is more difficult in the postmenopausal woman. For these estrogen-deficient women, using topical estrogen for a month, then repeating the examination may result in an adequate examination of the SCJ.

After visualizing the vagina, cervix, SCJ, the TZ, and cervical lesions, the areas must be assessed by close examination to determine clinical impression. The clinical impression will determine the biopsies taken. Size, shape, contour, and location of

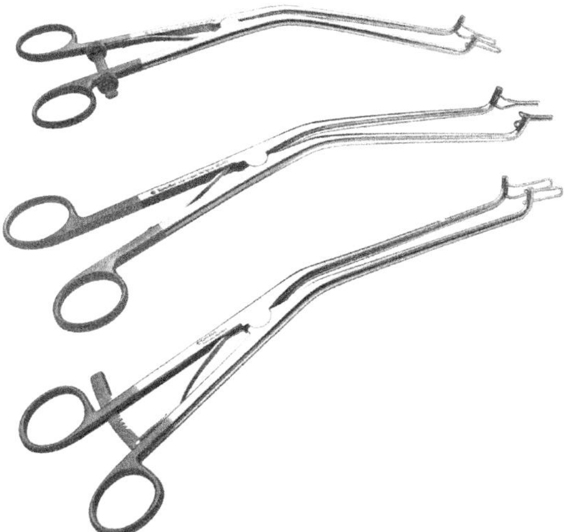

Fig. 5. Endocervical specula. (Product images provided courtesy of Cooper Surgical, Inc.)

the neoplasia will influence the selection of the appropriate treatment. Therefore, colposcopists should evaluate the lesions' characteristics while thinking about the treatment needed.

To predict the severity of the squamous disease, some colposcopists use an index like the Reid Colposcopic Index.[9] This index is based on 4 features: margin, color, vessels, and iodine staining (**Table 2**).[10] Others will use colposcopic features to differentiate normal from abnormal conditions. The colposcopist must be familiar with the terminology and the appearance of all normal and abnormal findings. A colposcopic atlas, training, and experience will facilitate learning about the features that are most important in differentiating normal from abnormal conditions.[4] The features considered most important are grouped systematically as follows:

1. *Epithelial Color*: before and after the application of normal saline, 3% to 5% acetic acid, or Lugol iodine solution.
2. *Vasculature*: type of vessel, vessel pattern, vessel caliber, and intercapillary distances.
3. *Surface Topography*: flat, ulcerated, or raised surfaces.
4. *Margin Characteristics*: border shape of the discrete epithelial lesions.

It must be stressed that no single colposcopic sign allows differentiation of the normal TZ from the abnormal one. These features and patterns must be studied and understood to describe the lower genital tract and to biopsy appropriate areas.[8] Although both methods are designed to help the colposcopist formulate a clinical impression to guide biopsies, it must be emphasized that more biopsies are likely better to detect higher-grade dysplasia.[11,12] Studies now document that the sensitivity of colposcopy for CIN 3 can be improved significantly by taking 2 or more biopsies.[13,14]

CERVICAL BIOPSY

After full evaluation of the size, shape, contour, location, and extent of the lesions, biopsies may then be taken. Most colposcopists begin with sampling the area of

Table 2
Modified Reid Colposcopic Index

Features	0 Points	1 Point	2 Points
Margin	Condylomatous Feathered margins Angular, jagged Satellite lesions Extend beyond transformation zone	Regular, smooth, straight	Rolled, peeling Internal demarcations
Color	Shiny, snow-white, indistinct	Shiny gray	Dull, oyster-white
Vessels	Fine-caliber Poorly formed patterns	Absent vessels	Punctuation or mosaic
Iodine	Positive staining Minor iodine negativity	Partial uptake	Negative staining of lesion
Sum of points with higher score more suggestive of dysplasia	0–2 CIN 1	3–4 CIN 1 or 2	5–8 CIN 2–3

Data from Chase DM, Kalouyan M, DiSaia PJ. Colposcopy to evaluate abnormal cervical cytology in 2008. Am J Obstet Gynecol 2009;200(5):472–80.

greatest concern for high-grade dysplasia or cancer. Sampling a specific area is best done under direct visualization through the colposcope. A sharp cervical biopsy forceps is usually placed at the lesion with the fixed jaw of the biopsy forceps closest to the external os. At times of biopsy on the sides of the cervix or farther outside of the external os, the forceps may be turned 90° or upside down to facilitate a good angle for the biopsy forceps. With the forceps jaws flush against the lesion to be biopsied, the forceps can be squeezed and closed firmly to sample the cervix. Biopsies need to be only 2 mm deep to sample the squamous epithelium that will incorporate the 4 distinct layers of the cervix: the basal cell layer, the parabasal cell layer, the intermediate cell layer, and the superficial or stratum corneum layer.

Communication should be clear with the patient, letting her know when the biopsy will take place and what to expect. This prepares the patient and provides a good signal for the assistant to help. Sharp, well-functioning biopsy forceps provide for a quick, smooth bite of the tissue without slipping or gnawing. The assistant can then take the biopsy forceps and remove the biopsy specimen from the jaws of the forceps with small pick-ups or teased out of the jaws with a broken wooden stick from a small cotton tip applicator. The colposcopist must confirm a good biopsy and the area of the biopsy should be reexamined to confirm that the biopsy was taken from the intended location. If there is significant bleeding from the site like may occur in pregnancy or with cervical cancer, a large cotton swab is immediately placed on the site to apply pressure and thus prevent "welling-up" of blood within the vagina. Additional biopsies are taken in appropriate areas.

Either silver nitrate sticks or cotton tip applicators filled with Monsel solution are applied to the biopsy site and its edges to provide hemostasis. If a bloody surface is present, a cotton swab is used to remove excess blood, then one of the agents is applied to the site. Rarely will bleeding be excessive. If bleeding is excessive, apply pressure to the exact site of bleeding while removing excess blood. The silver nitrate or Monsel solution can be reapplied and held with pressure for a few minutes. Very rarely will a stitch or packing in the vagina be needed, but these should be kept on hand for that rare instance.

Colposcopic biopsies are placed in pathology bottles containing fixative. Ideally, each specimen would be placed in a separate container marked with the exact location from which the biopsy was obtained. As some laboratories will charge according to the number of specimens received, the practitioner will need to decide whether to send the specimens in individual containers or to send the biopsies in the same container with clear documentation. The cervical biopsies should be sent separately from the endocervical sampling (ECS).

ECS

ECS has been considered a standard part of the colposcopic examination in nonpregnant patients until more recently. Findings from the ASCUS-LSIL Triage Study (ALTS) showed that clinicians were highly variable in their use of ECS.[15,16] Although there have been multiple studies evaluating the utility of the ECS, the current indications for ECS are summarized in **Table 3**, as published in the latest ASCCP guidelines.[3,17]

A few key ideas should be emphasized. ECS should be done with any nonpregnant patient who has had previous treatment for dysplasia. When a patient has had previous treatment for cervical neoplasia, there is a greater potential for a "skip lesion" where the dysplasia may not be contiguous from the TZ to the endocervix. In addition,

Table 3
Endocervical sampling of the nonpregnant patient during colposcopy

Pap Test	Colposcopic Impression	Endocervical Sampling Recommendations
ASCUS	Adequate colposcopy and lesion identified No lesions on colposcopy Inadequate colposcopy	Acceptable Preferred Preferred
LSIL	Adequate colposcopy and lesion identified No lesion identified Inadequate colposcopy	Acceptable Preferred Preferred
ASC-H	For all nonpregnant patients	Acceptable
HSIL AGC	For all nonpregnant patients	Recommended
Any abnormal pap test and history of treatment for CIN	Adequate or inadequate colposcopy	Recommended

Abbreviations: AGC, atypical glandular cells; ASC-H, high-grade squamous intraepithelial lesion; ASCUS, atypical squamous cells of undetermined significance; CIN, cervical intraepithelial lesion; HSIL, high-grade squamous intraepithelial lesion; LSIL, low-grade squamous intraepithelial lesion.

Data from Wright TC Jr, Massad LS, Dunton CJ, et al. 2006 consensus guidelines for the management of women with cervical intraepithelial neoplasia or adenocarcinoma in situ. J Low Genit Tract Dis 2007;11(4):223–39; and Massad LS, Einstein MH, Huh WK, et al. 2012 updated consensus guidelines for the management of abnormal cervical cancer screening tests and cancer precursors. J Low Genit Tract Dis 2013;17(5 Suppl 1):S1–27.

less experienced colposcopists should perform ECS on almost all nonpregnant patients, whereas more experienced colposcopists can be more selective according to the ASCCP guidelines.

There is some debate about the order of ECS and cervical biopsies. Some will argue that an ECS obtained before a cervical biopsy is preferred, as a cervical biopsy might leave a fragment at the cervical os that will be picked up with the ECS, thus creating a false-positive specimen. Others want to biopsy the most concerning area first so as not to create bleeding that might obscure visibility. The vital aspect of ECS is obtaining an adequate specimen when needed.

Two options exist for sampling the endocervix: the endocervical curettage (ECC) and the endocervical brush. The endocervical curette should be held like a uterine curette and placed 1 to 2 cm into the cervix. With pressure on the handle of the curette so that the instrument is held like a fulcrum, the distal tip of the curette is pressed against the inside of the cervical canal and pulled toward the colposcopist to sample the endocervix in 360° of the canal. The curette should then be removed directly away from the endocervix to avoid contact with the ectocervix. To remove the specimen from the curette, the assistant can flush the tip of the curette in the specimen container. A forceps or a cervical brush can then be placed within the endocervical canal to remove additional biopsy fragments, ensuring a satisfactory sampling. The second option is to use only a cervical brush instead of a curette. The brush should be placed within the endocervical canal and rotated, vigorously moving the brush back and forth several millimeters. The cervical brush can then be removed and placed in a specimen container.

Although the ECC and the endocervical brush seem to produce equivalent amounts of tissue and cells, the brush seems to have a greater sensitivity but a higher false-positive rate. The ECC has greater specificity of disease than the cervical brush.[18,19]

For some menopausal patients or patients with cervical stenosis, the cervical brush seems to be easier to use and acceptable.[20]

DOCUMENTATION FOR COLPOSCOPY

Documentation of the colposcopy should include the pertinent history, colposcopic findings, colposcopic impression, and management plans. Using a standardized form facilitates complete and accurate documentation for the record (see Appendix A). A diagram of the vulva and cervix allows for easy diagramming of the anatomic findings. Simple abbreviations can be used on the diagram, including marking of the external os, the location of the SCJ, and the colposcopic findings and/or lesions found. Additional symbols like an "X" are used to mark where biopsies were taken. The adequacy of the colposcopy should be recorded followed by the impression and plan. On many occasions, the plan will include awaiting the histology results.

POSTCOLPOSCOPIC INSTRUCTIONS

Following colposcopy, patients need to know what was found on the examination and what can be said about the findings. In most cases, an experienced colposcopist can communicate a clinical impression and appropriately reassure the patient if there is no evidence of cancer. The exact diagnosis will be pending but patients strongly desire to know what can be known after the examination. Setting expectations with clear communication of when the patient will be notified with results is important and will depend on the laboratory used.

It is recommended to give both verbal and written instructions following colposcopy. Sanitary pads should be offered to the patient following colposcopy. Most practitioners will recommend abstaining from sexual activity for several days to prevent possible bleeding from the biopsy sites. NSAIDs may be given to the patient if needed and can be taken at home for pelvic pain or uterine cramping. The patient should be informed that mild vaginal bleeding with or without a vaginal discharge from the silver nitrate or Monsel solution is common for several days. Heavy bleeding more than a normal menstrual cycle, increased pain, or foul discharge should prompt a call to the office.

SUMMARY FOR COLPOSCOPY

Colposcopy requires knowledge, experience, judgment, skill, and expertise. Although knowledge of the procedure is essential, great understanding is required concerning the anatomy of the lower genital tract, indications for colposcopy, assessment of findings, correlation of cytologic and histologic findings, and options for management. Structured training and guidance are essential to develop skills with dexterity and proficiency with the procedure, while providing excellent patient care. Significant experience and ongoing education will prevent errors, while providing effective and appropriate patient care. The goal of the colposcopic examination will be met when the source of the abnormal cells on Pap test are identified, the type and grade of the lesion(s) are diagnosed, and the approach to treatment is determined.

LOOP ELECTROSURGICAL EXCISION PROCEDURE

Treatment methods for CIN are categorized as ablative methods that destroy the affected cervical tissue in vivo and excisional methods that remove the affected tissue. Ablative methods include cryotherapy, laser ablation, electrofulguration, and cold coagulation. Excisional methods include cold-knife conization (CKC), loop electrosurgical excision procedure (LEEP), laser conization, and electrosurgical needle conization. Excisional methods are widely used, as they provide a tissue specimen for pathologic examination, but there is no overwhelming superior technique for eradicating CIN.[21] The choice of treatment of ectocervical lesions must be based on cost, morbidity, and whether an excisional treatment provides more reliable specimen for assessment of disease compared with colposcopic biopsy then treatment with an ablation method. LEEP is an excisional method performed in the office that is cheaper than other excisional methods and requires less expertise than other excisional procedures. This article focuses on the proper use of LEEP as a procedure in the management of CIN.

Electrosurgery has been around for almost a century. It was first introduced in the 1920s by William Bovie and Harvey Cushing.[4] In the early 1980s, large loop excision of the transformation zone (LLETZ) was introduced into clinical practice in the United Kingdom using high-frequency energy for surgical cutting and hemostasis. LEEP was later termed in the early 1990s in North America to refer to a similar procedure using smaller electrodes.

Traditionally, LEEP is performed following colposcopy and biopsy-confirmed CIN. In this approach, diagnosis and treatment occur at 2 different visits. Hence, the diagnosis of CIN is confirmed with colposcopy and biopsy, then the LEEP serves as the treatment of the lesion.

There are instances when the surgeon may perform diagnosis and treatment during the same visit, referred to as the "see-and-treat" approach. The "see-and-treat" approach should be considered only after cytology-confirmed high-grade squamous intraepithelial lesion (HGSIL), a colposcopic examination that reveals lesions concerning for dysplasia, and informed consent that the patient would prefer this approach.[4] The primary benefit of this approach is convenience facilitating 1 clinic visit in patients who are at high risk for CIN 2 or greater lesions or if a patient is not expected to be compliant with follow-up visits. The "see-and-treat" approach should not be used in adolescents, young women, LSIL, ASC-US, ASC-H, or AGC.

Indications

LEEP is indicated per guidelines,[3] including the following clinical scenarios: (1) when it is necessary to remove the TZ; (2) when treatment for CIN is required per guidelines; (3) when colposcopy is inadequate with ASC-H or HSIL pap test; (4) when dysplasia involves the endocervical canal or when the ECC shows CIN; and (5) when microinvasion is suspected and pathologic diagnosis is needed. LEEP should be considered in instances in which there is discrepancy between cytology, colposcopy, and histology findings, especially if high-grade dysplasia is suspected.

Clinicians should consider several factors when deciding if LEEP is the appropriate procedure. These factors include the patient's age, parity, pregnancy status, and prior cervical cytology. Special circumstances should apply to adolescents and women 24 years and younger.[3] In addition, the clinician must be able to competently perform the procedure and appropriately manage complications that might arise with the procedure.

Contraindications to LEEP include an uncooperative patient, presence of cervical inflammatory process, obvious cancer, pregnancy, bleeding disorders, or Diethylstilbestrol (DES) abnormality. There are some instances in which a CKC may be preferable over a LEEP. These instances occur when a deep cone specimen is preferred without a central burn margin, when glandular disease is documented by colposcopic-guided biopsy, or when microinvasive disease is suspected.[4] The CKC gives less burn artifact and allows for staging of cancer.

Patient Counseling and Preparation

It is optimal for the patient to be familiar with the practitioner performing the LEEP. A review of the patient's history, similar to a colposcopy history, should be completed. A pregnancy test should be performed to exclude pregnancy if needed. Consent, preferably in written form, explaining the indications, risks, benefits, and alternatives should be obtained, allowing the patient to become familiar with the process. The practitioner should confirm patient understanding and answer questions as needed. The great benefits of LEEP are allowing the provider to obtain a tissue specimen for diagnosis and treatment of CIN while obviating the need to take patients to the operating room using general anesthesia.

Immediate risks and long-term consequences of LEEP should be reviewed. The most common complication is a 4% to 6% risk of bleeding, which rarely requires hospitalization to manage.[4] Other minor risks include pain, infection, and damage to the vaginal sidewalls. In the long term, LEEP may result in an increased risk of adverse pregnancy outcomes, including preterm delivery, low birth weight, and premature rupture of membranes. A 2006 review of the literature by Kyrgiou and colleagues[22] found that LLETZ was associated with a significant increase in the risk of preterm delivery (Relative risk [RR] 1.70; confidence interval [CI] 1.24–2.35), low birth weight (RR 1.82; CI 1.09–3.06), and preterm premature rupture of membranes (RR1.26; CI 1.62–4.46). They found no significant difference in the risk of cesarean delivery, neonatal intensive care unit admission, or perinatal mortality. More recently, in a retrospective study of 511 women who delivered with a preceding LEEP procedure, no evidence of increased risk of preterm birth or significant associations with perinatal mortality were found.[23]

The importance of an appropriately functioning colposcope and proper set-up for LEEP equipment cannot be overemphasized. It is often necessary to perform a colposcopic examination to examine the cervix before LEEP. Equipment needed to perform the LEEP include the following:

- Colposcope
- 3% to 5% acetic acid solution or Lugol solution
- Insulated specula of various sizes
- Various sizes of loop electrodes
- 3-mm to 5-mm ball electrode
- Local anesthetic plus vasoconstrictor solution (1%–2% lidocaine with 1:100,000 epinephrine)
- 27-gauge Potocky or lumbar puncture needle with 10-mL syringe
- Small and large cotton swabs
- Electrosurgical generator
- Grounding pad
- Smoke evacuator system
- Smoke evacuation tubing
- Monsel solution
- Safety masks and goggles for the clinician

Electrosurgery uses radiofrequency current to cut or coagulate tissue. The basic principles for electrosurgery are that (1) electricity flows to the ground, (2) electricity will follow the path of least resistance, and (3) impedance to electric current produces heat.[4] As human tissue, or the cervix in this case, resists the flow of electrical current, the impedance will create heat required to cut or coagulate the tissue. A good understanding of electrosurgical principles is highly recommended. Electrosurgery requires high voltage, high frequency, and low current density. Vaporization of tissue results in cutting, whereas dehydration of tissue results in coagulation, desiccation, and fulguration.

The electrosurgical system has 3 components: the electrosurgical generator, the active electrode (the loop or roller ball), and the patient return pad or dispersive electrode (the grounding pad placed on the patient's thigh). The alternating current flows from the electrosurgical generator to the active electrode (Loop or rollerball) at the cervix and back through the patient to the patient return pad or dispersive electrode on the patient (**Fig. 6**). Most modern electrosurgical generators will use a return electrode monitoring system designed to reduce or eliminate the risks of burns on the patient at the site of the dispersive electrode. There are a variety of LEEP systems available to clinicians, often being portable and integrating the electrosurgical generator, the smoke evacuation unit, and internal storage (**Fig. 7**). Assorted features for the equipment include hand or foot controls as well as pure sine waveform for cutting or blended waveform modes for a more hemostatic effect.

Regardless of the electrosurgical generator chosen, it is important for the clinician to be familiar with basic electrosurgical principles and the function of the electrosurgical unit before performing a LEEP on patients. Some clinicians may find it beneficial to use simulation to practice a LEEP on items such as hot dogs, peaches, or chicken so as to familiarize oneself with the equipment and to review technique and electrosurgical principles. New LEEP surgeons should seek opportunities for preceptorships with experienced LEEP surgeons. The ASCCP offers courses on LEEPs for practitioners.

A variety of specula are available for LEEP procedures. The specula must be nonconductive and, ideally, have an attachment for a disposable smoke evacuator tubing (**Fig. 8**). The Occupational Safety and Health Administration requires a smoke evacuator to reduce exposure to the odors and possible viral-laden smoke produced by LEEP. Nonconductive, insulated specula are required to prevent transmission of electric current through the walls of the patient's vagina. Insulated specula vary in size and shapes and are available in Graves and Pedersen designs. If needed, nonconductive vaginal sidewall retractors can be placed before the speculum to improve visualization by retracting redundant tissue laterally and to reduce the risk of thermal injury to the vagina. Most of these instruments are autoclavable for sterilization.

There is an assortment of loop electrodes available for clinicians that come in different shapes, widths, and depths (**Fig. 9**). Electrodes are usually composed of an oval or square loop attached to an insulated shaft. Loop electrodes range in size from approximately 0.4 cm deep and 1.0 cm wide to 1.0 cm deep and 2.0 cm wide.

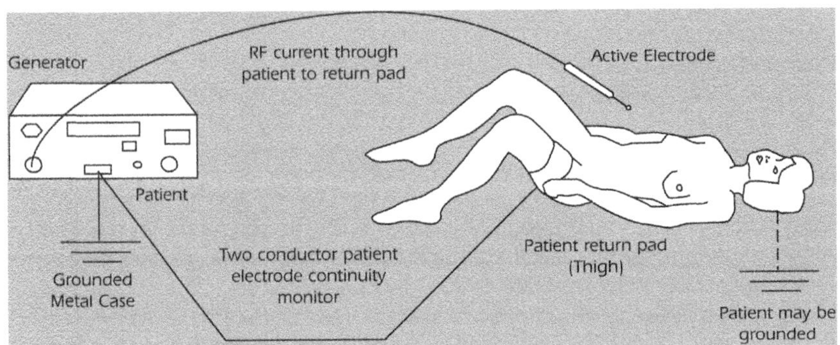

Fig. 6. LEEP set-up with electrosurgical generator, active electrode and patient return pad. (Product images provided courtesy of Cooper Surgical, Inc.)

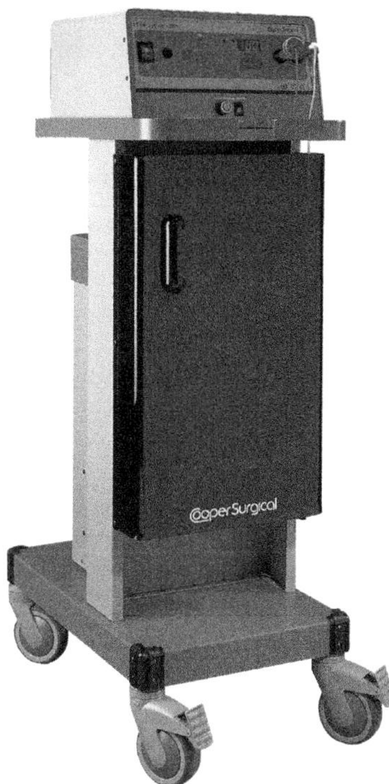

Fig. 7. Portable LEEP system with electrosurgical generator, smoke evacuator, and internal storage. (Product images provided courtesy of Cooper Surgical, Inc.)

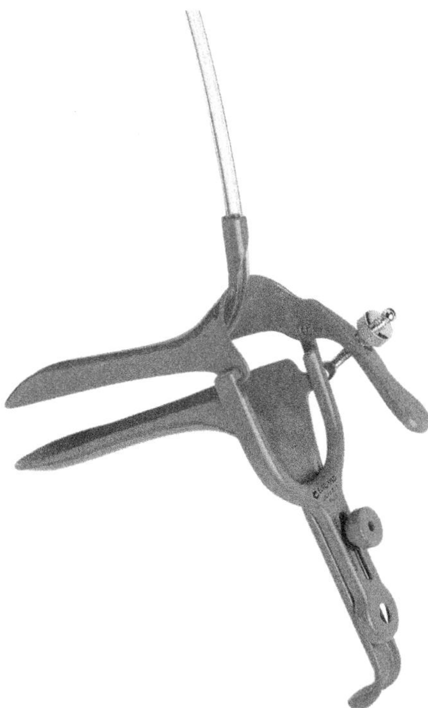

Fig. 8. Insulated speculum with vacuum tubing. (Product images provided courtesy of Cooper Surgical, Inc.)

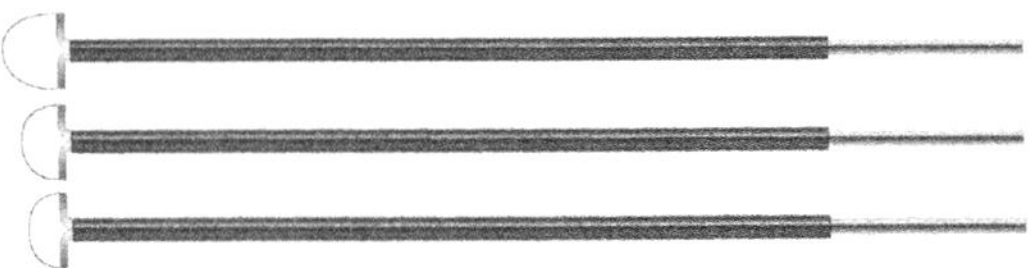

Fig. 9. Sample of assorted loops for loop electrosurgical excision procedures. (Product images provided courtesy of Cooper Surgical, Inc.)

Ball electrodes are available in 3-mm or 5-mm size to perform fulguration of the cone bed after loop excision.

Several options are available for local anesthetics; 1% lidocaine with epinephrine is commonly used as local anesthetic. The addition of epinephrine offers a vasoconstrictor benefit that assists with minimizing bleeding. Some providers use vasopressin instead of epinephrine. Providers should inform patients that injection of epinephrine or vasopressin is likely to increase their heart rate, resulting in the sensation that their heart is racing. Optimally, the equipment will be completely set up with materials readily available before the patient enters the procedure room.

Procedure

The patient should be positioned on the examination table in dorsal lithotomy position with feet in stirrups. The dispersive pad should be placed on the patient's thigh as close as possible to the cervix. Performing a bimanual examination allows the physician to assess the size of the uterus, position of the cervix, and presence or absence of uterine tenderness. An insulated speculum, with attached suction tubing, should be placed in the vagina and the cervix should be centered in the visual field. If the vaginal side walls have excess laxity and there is concern for thermal injury, an insulated vaginal sidewall retractor can be used. Alternatively, a glove or condom can be cut and placed around the speculum before insertion into the vagina, which will function to hold the vaginal side walls out of the operative field. Adequate exposure and visualization of the cervix before starting the excision is fundamental. The cervix should be perpendicular to the long axis of the vagina. Colposcopy should be performed to identify the TZ, the SCJ, and the extent of the lesion; 3% to 5% acetic acid or Lugol solution can be applied to highlight the abnormal areas for excision.

With good patient communication, the local anesthetic with vasoconstrictor solution (usually $\leq$10 mL) should be injected intracervically at the 3, 6, 9, and 12 o'clock positions 2 to 4 mm below the mucosal surface until good blanching occurs. After the initial injection, placement of the needle at the lateral aspects of the blanched cervical mucosa will minimize the number of "sticks" that the patient will feel. Sometimes, more than 4 injections will be needed to anesthetize the cervix appropriately.

The electrosurgical unit should be set to the recommended power setting for loop excision as advised by the manufacturer. Most LEEP surgeons prefer to use the cutting mode, whereas others like the blended mode. The cutting mode produces less burn artifact, as there is less lateral spread of electric current. A pass with the cutting mode is also less likely to stick with the LEEP procedure. The blended mode is better with coagulation of vessels and can reduce bleeding in some settings. The blended mode is best for coagulation of bleeding sites using fulguration with the ball electrode following removal of the LEEP specimen.

In selecting the technical approach, the LEEP surgeon has several options depending on the size and location of the cervical neoplasia. The 2011 International Federation of Cervical Pathology and Colposcopy Colposcopic Terminology of the Cervix classifies the TZ into types 1, 2, and 3 in relation to the visibility of the SCJ. Using this classification facilitates communication and documentation. The type 1 TZ refers to situations in which the SCJ can be seen in its entirety. Type 2 refers to instances in which the SCJ is partially visible. Type 3 refers to circumstances in which the SCJ is not visible.[8]

The goal for the diagnosis or treatment for the individual patient needs to be kept in mind: to eradicate the neoplasia by removing the smallest volume of tissue. Three basic approaches are used: (1) to remove the ectocervix only; (2) to remove the endocervix only; or (3) to remove the ectocervix followed by a second pass of the endocervix removing a "top hat" portion the cervix. A "top hat" is a narrower loop excision that allows the clinician to remove the inner portion of the endocervical canal.

For removal of the ectocervix, the LEEP surgeon should select the loop size that would remove the dysplastic tissue and TZ in one pass. Some surgeons perform a LEEP under visualization through the colposcope whereas others operate under direct visualization. Knowing the exact location of the disease makes either approach acceptable. There are instances in which it may be necessary to make multiple passes to facilitate removal of a wider lesion or TZ. This planning and visualization of the procedure with selection of the best loop will mitigate problems with the LEEP. The selected loop is placed in the hand piece with the colposcopist confirming that the loop will pass easily within speculum and vaginal side walls. It may be helpful to rehearse or "ghost" the movement to ensure easy and adequate excision while avoiding contact with the vaginal sidewalls. Sometimes, a large, moistened cotton swab or a wooden tongue depressor is placed in the lateral fornix to protect the vaginal side wall or to provide a better angle to perform the LEEP.

The circuit setup should be confirmed, the patient should be informed of the noises she will hear, and the vacuum aspirator should be activated by the assistant. The LEEP surgeon may begin at the 9, 12, 3, or 6 o'clock position. The choice of where to begin depends on the extent of the lesion and the comfort of the LEEP surgeon. The top of the loop is placed just outside of the area to be excised; the current is activated by the foot pedal or button on the hand piece; and the loop is moved smoothly into and across the cervix, allowing the current to cut the tissue. The technique involves one continuous movement lasting about 5 seconds taking care to ensure the loop is free from vaginal sidewalls when activated. The depth of the excision should be 7 to 10 mm, as 86% of CIN 3 will have a depth of 10 mm or less.[4] When moving the loop at the appropriate speed, the current will cut through the cervix without resistance or obstruction to the activated wire. The current remains on during the excision until the loop is removed from the cervix. The specimen should be removed with forceps and set aside. When multiple passes are necessary, the area with the highest-grade dysplasia should be removed first. Additional passes are made as needed.

Excision of the endocervix alone is useful for lesions that are confined to the endocervical canal. The removal of the endocervix is best done with a loop that is narrower with more depth to the loop (see **Fig. 9**). The endocervical LEEP is performed in a similar fashion. If there is concern about dysplasia above the endocervical LEEP pass, an ECC can be performed following the LEEP, with this specimen sent in a separate pathology container.

For lesions that extend beyond 10 mm in depth into the os, the combined extocervical and endocervical "top hat" approach is preferred. The LEEP surgeon should choose the loops with this plan in mind. The ectocervix should be removed in one pass with a wider and shallower loop. The endocervix can then be excised with a narrower, deeper loop.

There are times when the LEEP surgeon needs to troubleshoot during the procedure. Occasionally, the loop may become stuck due to tissue impedance, the loop breaking, exposure becoming suboptimal, or pain requiring more local anesthesia. In these instances, the procedure should be stopped and the problem fixed. The LEEP can then be restarted from the same angle or the excision can be done from the opposite side working toward the point where the electrode was stuck.

After the excision, the setting on the electrosurgical unit should be switched to the blended or coagulation mode. Blood should be removed or dabbed with a cotton swab. The ball electrode is used to fulgurate the bleeding sites at the cone bed and edges of the LEEP. With fulguration, the ball electrode is held a few millimeters from the tissue and the spark travels across the tissue gap from the ball to the cervix, providing coagulation via superficial dehydration of the tissue.

After good hemostasis is obtained, the ball electrode and speculum are removed from the vagina. The patient should remain supine until she feels comfortable with sitting. While the patient recovers, the surgeon may label the specimen(s) by tagging to show the anatomic orientation. The specimen(s) should then be placed in formalin and sent to pathology.

Postprocedure Care After LEEP

Patients may be offered NSAIDs to alleviate with pain. Providers should discuss precautions and reasons to seek medical advice. These include heavy vaginal bleeding, abnormal malodorous discharge, or severe abdominal pain. Patients should be advised to avoid sexual intercourse or using tampons or vaginal douche products for approximately 2 weeks after LEEP. A follow-up appointment should be scheduled in 2 to 4 weeks to review pathology and plan for further evaluation per guidelines.[3]

PERFORMING CRYOTHERAPY

The use of cryotherapy gained popularity in the 1970s, providing the first outpatient treatment option for CIN. Cryotherapy destroys pathologic tissue of the cervix by freezing the tissue. Before this time, CKC or hysterectomy were the preferred treatments. Today, a variety of methods for treatment of CIN are available with 2 basic options. Ablative procedures include cryotherapy, laser vaporization, and cold coagulation of the cervix. Excisional procedures include LEEP or LLETZ, laser conization, CKC, and hysterectomy.

LEEP procedures have become preferred in most settings because of the ease of office treatment; and as an excisional procedure, it removes tissue, allowing for examination of the specimen to identify occult carcinoma. When selecting the treatment for CIN, the procedure chosen should be the one that offers the best cure rate considering the lesion's characteristics and the clinician's expertise. Studies comparing all of the treatment options have been small and have had difficulties distinguishing subtle differences among the treatments.[21,24] The 2012 World Health Organization expert panel recommends LEEP over cryotherapy when LEEP is available and accessible but recommends cryotherapy over no treatment.[25]

Therefore, although LEEP is preferred, cryotherapy continues to be popular because of the lower skill required, minimal complications, and cost-effectiveness. Cryotherapy is effective and appropriate when used with strict adherence to treatment guidelines. This article focuses on the proper technique using cryotherapy.

Indications

The ASCCP has published consensus guidelines for management of abnormal cervical cancer screening tests and cancer precursors.[3] In general, and with an adequate colposcopy, cryotherapy can be used with persistent CIN 1 for at least 2 years or with high-grade CIN (CIN 2, CIN 3, or CIN 2,3). A diagnostic excisional procedure is recommended for women with recurrent high-grade CIN.

The objectives of cryotherapy of the cervix are as follows: (1) to prevent the progression of CIN to cervical cancer, (2) to expose all CIN tissue to lethal temperatures, (3) to destroy the entire TZ, (4) to protect surrounding normal lower genital tract tissue from injury, and (5) to minimize treatment side effects of patient discomfort and complications.[4]

Cryotherapy should be used only after rigorous exclusion of invasive cancer. The presence of cancer must be excluded by means of prior assessments with cytology, colposcopy, and histology. Colposcopic guidelines for the use of cryotherapy necessitate (1) adequate colposcopy with visualization of the entire squamocolumnar junction; (2) visualization of the entire lesion(s); (3) consistent cytologic and colposcopic findings; and (4) absence of endocervical neoplasia as documented by a negative ECC, a negative cytobrush endocervical sampling, or a normal satisfactory endocervical colposcopy.[4] The lesion must be smaller than 75% of the cervix, as the cryotip should cover the lesion and the largest cryotip typically covers only lesions that extend up to 75% of the cervix.[26] Also, the lesion must not extend into the endocervical canal by more than 3 to 4 mm.[4]

Contraindications for cryotherapy include (1) invasive cervical cancer, (2) pregnancy, (3) in utero DES exposure, (4) acute cervicitis, (5) cryoglobulinemia, (6) positive ECC, (7) unsatisfactory colposcopy, (8) lesions larger than 75% of the cervix, (9) lesions that extend more than 5 mm into the endocervical canal, and (10) exophytic, nodular, or papillary lesions or an obstetric scar that hinders proper application of the cryoprobe to the cervix and TZ.[4] With strict adherence to these objectives, requirements, and contraindications, cryotherapy can be used appropriately (**Table 4**).

Patient Counseling and Preparation

Before cryotherapy, the patient should be screened for *Chlamydia trachomatis* and *Neisseria gonorrhoeae* if indicated. The best time to perform cryotherapy is immediately after a normal menstrual cycle. A urine pregnancy test should be performed if needed. NSAID medications may be taken 1 hour before cryotherapy to minimize pain. An intracervical block or paracervical block with local anesthesia may be used to further reduce discomfort but is not required. The size and distribution of the lesion must have been delineated colposcopically to ensure its appropriate use.

Patients should then be counseled and consented about the indications for cryotherapy, particularly the guidelines for ablative therapy and the risks, benefits, and options of CIN management available. Patients should understand that cryotherapy causes a "burn" with the freezing of the cervix and the patient may experience mild to moderate menstrual cramping during the procedure. Following treatment, the patient will have a watery and occasionally blood-tinged, malodorous discharge for 2 to 4 weeks.

Equipment for cryotherapy includes gloves, a vaginal speculum, vaginal side wall retractors (if needed), large cotton swabs, water soluble gel, Monsel paste, the compressed gas cylinder with a pressure gauge on the regulator, a cryogun attached via a line to the gas cylinder (**Fig. 10**), cryoprobe tips in various shapes/sizes, and a timer to record time of freezing. Several different cryogens can be used for cryotherapy with the most common being nitrous oxide and carbon dioxide. Practitioners must be fully trained in the use of the equipment with special care taken for monitoring the pressure in the cylinders, storage of gas cylinders, and maintenance of the cryogun. The cryogun is activated by depressing the button or trigger on the gun and can often be locked in place during the procedure. The defrost is activated by releasing the

Table 4
Objectives, guidelines, and contraindications for cryotherapy

Objectives for cryotherapy	Prevent the progression of CIN to cervical cancer Expose all CIN to tissue lethal temperatures Destroy the entire transformation zone Protect surrounding normal lower genital tract tissue from injury Minimize treatment side effects of patient discomfort and complications.
Requirements for cryotherapy use	Adequate colposcopy with visualization of the entire SCJ Visualization of the entire lesion(s) Consistent cytologic and colposcopic findings Absence of endocervical neoplasia as documented by • A negative ECC • A negative cytobrush endocervical sampling, or • A normal satisfactory endocervical colposcopy The lesion must be smaller than 75% of the cervix Lesion not extending into the endocervical canal more than 3–4 mm
Contraindications for cryotherapy	Invasive cervical cancer Pregnancy In utero diethylstilbestrol (DES) exposure Acute cervacitis Cryoglobulinemia Positive ECC Unsatisfactory colposcopy Lesions larger than 75% of the cervix Lesions that extend more than 5 mm into the endocervical canal[26,a] Exophytic, nodular, or papillary lesions or an obstetric scar that hinders proper application of the cryoprobe to the cervix and transformation zone

Abbreviations: CIN, cervical intraepithelial lesion; ECC, endocervical curettage; SCJ, squamocolumnar junction.

[a] In settings where excisional procedure or referral for additional treatment is not available, the World Health Organization expert panel suggests that women with lesions extending into the endocervical canal be treated with cryotherapy.

Data from Refs.[4,25,26]

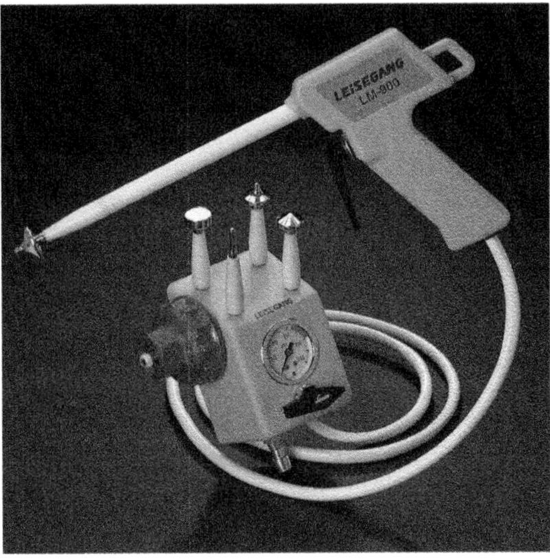

Fig. 10. Cryogun with pressure gauge. (Product images provided courtesy of Cooper Surgical, Inc.)

trigger or by depressing a separate defrost button that will thaw the cryotip rapidly. The practitioner can choose the size and shape of the cryotip based on the size of the cervix and size of the lesion to be treated. The most commonly used tips are 19 mm and 25 mm with the tips being either flat or cone-shaped (**Fig. 11**). Some tips will have a nipple-shaped tip designed to be placed at the external os. The entire lesion should be encompassed by the cryotip to avoid the need for treatment of areas outside the probe. If a lesion is not encompassed by the initial iceball, an additional application is required using the flat cryotip on the area outside the initially treated area.

Procedure

The patient should be positioned on an examination table in dorsal lithotomy position with feet in stirrups and a speculum placed with adequate visualization of the cervix. Wipe the cervix with a cotton swab soaked with acetic acid to outline the abnormality if needed. The best cryotip should be chosen and measured on the cervix to ensure that the cryoprobe will seat well on the cervix and cover the entire lesion. The lesion should not extend more than 2 mm beyond the probe for adequate treatment.[26] A film of water-soluble gel is applied to the probe, which allows smooth contact with the cervix and permits release of the probe tip from the cervix after freezing.[4] The cryotip is attached to the cryogun and the tip containing the gel is then seated on the cervix. Ensure that the cryoprobe is not in contact with surrounding vaginal walls. If needed, the practitioner may use a vaginal side wall retractor, a tongue blade, a large cotton swab, or a condom/glove placed over the speculum to protect the vaginal walls from being inadvertently touched with the frozen probe tip. Remind the patient that she might feel some discomfort or cramping while you are freezing the cervix.

With the cryotip in the center of the cervical os, a timer is set and the cryogun should be activated, which will cause the cryotip to adhere to the cervix. Once the iceball is formed, firmer pressure on the cryoprobe or gentle traction with the cryogun will straighten the cervix within the vaginal canal, providing a larger safe zone surrounding the freezing probe. The World Health Organization (WHO) recommends 2 cycles of freezing and thawing: 3 minutes freezing, followed by 5 minutes thawing, followed by a further 3 minutes freezing.[26]

Cryotherapy works via the concept in physics of heat transfer in which heat is removed from the cervix to the cryoprobe. It is felt that a rapid freeze with a slow

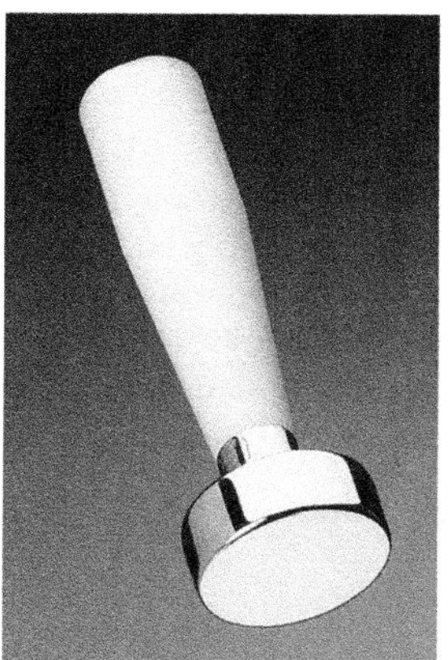
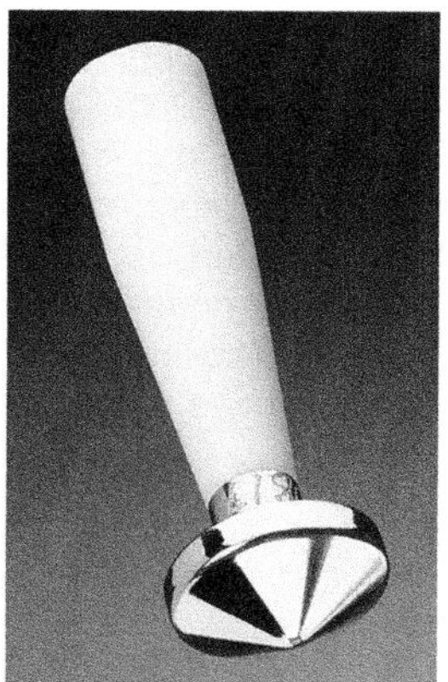
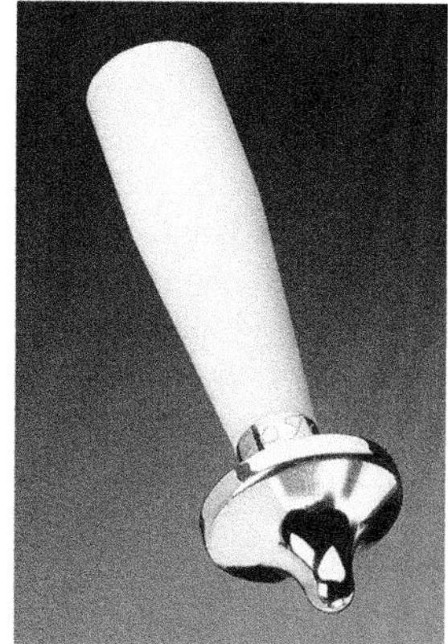

Fig. 11. Cryotherapy tips. (Product images provided courtesy of Cooper Surgical, Inc.)

defrost is the most the most effective means of inducing tissue damage.[4] Following the first 3-minute freeze, the cervix will usually defrost over the 5-minute thawing period. If the cryogun has a defrost feature, it can be initiated by squeezing this button several times. When thawed, gently rotate the probe on the cervix to dislodge and remove it. Removing the cryoprobe before it is fully thawed can pull tissue off the cervix. The TZ is examined to ensure the probe was well positioned over the intended treatment area.

Before the second freeze, the cervix should "thaw" from an icy white appearance to the normal pink color. The second 3-minute freeze should then be performed in a similar fashion. When the second freezing is completed, allow time for thawing of the probe or use the defrost button before attempting to remove the probe from the cervix. The probe can then be removed, leaving the area you have frozen appearing white. If there are larger lesions or a TZ that was not completely covered, overlapping applications of the cryoprobe may be done to ensure complete treatment of all areas. The cervix should be examined for bleeding. If needed, Monsel paste may be applied. The speculum can then be removed.

Postprocedure Care

The patient should be given a sanitary pad if needed and counseled to expect 2 to 4 weeks of a watery, vaginal discharge that may be malodorous, blood-tinged, and profuse. NSAIDs are used for pain and uterine cramping following the procedure. Patients should abstain from intercourse and not use tampons until the discharge resolves. WHO recommends that patients return in 2 to 6 weeks for examination,[26] whereas other authorities state that postsurgical follow-up is not necessary unless complications arise.[4] Either way, the patient should return sooner if she develops a fever with temperature higher than 38°C, shaking chills, severe lower abdominal pain, foul-smelling or puslike discharge, or bleeding for more than 2 days or bleeding with clots.[26]

Following the procedure, the cryoprobe should be cleaned and disinfected per manufacturer recommendations. It is critical that the hollow part of the cryotip is completely dry when used next or the water inside the probe will freeze and the probe could crack or the treatment not work. The cryotherapy unit, hose, and regulator should be decontaminated by wiping them with alcohol. Proper use, cleaning, and disinfecting are essential for safe use in cryotherapy.[26]

With strict use of guidelines, appropriate counseling of patients, and proper technique in the office, cryotherapy is an effective, acceptable, and safe outpatient treatment for CIN. Cure rates after treatment with cryotherapy range from 85% to 94%.[27] The effectiveness of cryotherapy is comparable to CKC biopsy (90%–94%), laser conization (93%–96%), LEEP (91%–98%), and laser ablation (95%–96%).[21] As there is a 5% to 15% risk of residual disease in women treated with cryotherapy, long-term follow-up should include cotesting with a Pap test and HPV typing at 12 and 24 months per current guidelines.[3] If both cotests are negative, retesting in 3 years is acceptable. If one of the tests is abnormal, repeat colposcopy with endocervical sampling is recommended. If all tests are negative, routine screening is recommended for at least 20 years.

REFERENCES

1. Emmert F. The recognition of cancer of the uterus in its earliest stages. JAMA 1931;97.

2. Townsend DE, Morrow CP, editors. Synopsis of gynecologic oncology. 2nd edition. New York: Wiley, John & Sons, Incorporated; 1981.
3. Massad LS, Einstein MH, Huh WK, et al. 2012 updated consensus guidelines for the management of abnormal cervical cancer screening tests and cancer precursors. J Low Genit Tract Dis 2013;17(5 Suppl 1):S1–27.
4. Mayeaux EJ, Cox TJ, editors. Modern colposcopy textbook and atlas. 3rd edition. Philadelphia: Wolters Kluwer/Lippincott Williams and Wilkins; 2012.
5. Gajjar K, Martin-Hirsch PP, Bryant A. Pain relief for women with cervical intraepithelial neoplasia undergoing colposcopy treatment. Cochrane Database Syst Rev 2012;(10):CD006120.
6. Church L, Oliver L, Dobie S, et al. Analgesia for colposcopy: double-masked, randomized comparison of ibuprofen and benzocaine gel. Obstet Gynecol 2001; 97(1):5–10.
7. Swancutt DR, Greenfield SM, Wilson S. Women's colposcopy experience and preferences: a mixed methods study. BMC Womens Health 2008;8:2.
8. Bornstein J, Bentley J, Bosze P, et al. 2011 colposcopic terminology of the International Federation for Cervical Pathology and Colposcopy. Obstet Gynecol 2012;120(1):166–72.
9. Reid R, Campion MJ. HPV-associated lesions of the cervix: biology and colposcopic features. Clin Obstet Gynecol 1989;32(1):157–79.
10. Chase DM, Kalouyan M, DiSaia PJ. Colposcopy to evaluate abnormal cervical cytology in 2008. Am J Obstet Gynecol 2009;200(5):472–80.
11. Cox JT. More questions about the accuracy of colposcopy: what does this mean for cervical cancer prevention? Obstet Gynecol 2008;111(6):1266–7.
12. Pretorius RG, Belinson JL, Burchette RJ, et al. Regardless of skill, performing more biopsies increases the sensitivity of colposcopy. J Low Genit Tract Dis 2011;15(3):180–8.
13. Gage JC, Hanson VW, Abbey K, et al. Number of cervical biopsies and sensitivity of colposcopy. Obstet Gynecol 2006;108(2):264–72.
14. Pretorius RG, Zhang WH, Belinson JL, et al. Colposcopically directed biopsy, random cervical biopsy, and endocervical curettage in the diagnosis of cervical intraepithelial neoplasia II or worse. Am J Obstet Gynecol 2004;191(2):430–4.
15. ASCUS-LSIL Triage Study (ALTS) Group. Results of a randomized trial on the management of cytology interpretations of atypical squamous cells of undetermined significance. Am J Obstet Gynecol 2003;188(6):1383–92.
16. Solomon D, Stoler M, Jeronimo J, et al. Diagnostic utility of endocervical curettage in women undergoing colposcopy for equivocal or low-grade cytologic abnormalities. Obstet Gynecol 2007;110(2 Pt 1):288–95.
17. Wright TC Jr, Massad LS, Dunton CJ, et al. 2006 consensus guidelines for the management of women with cervical intraepithelial neoplasia or adenocarcinoma in situ. J Low Genit Tract Dis 2007;11(4):223–39.
18. Gibson CA, Trask CE, House P, et al. Endocervical sampling: a comparison of endocervical brush, endocervical curette, and combined brush with curette techniques. J Low Genit Tract Dis 2001;5(1):1–6.
19. Hoffman MS, Sterghos S Jr, Gordy LW, et al. Evaluation of the cervical canal with the endocervical brush. Obstet Gynecol 1993;82(4 Pt 1):573–7.
20. Martin D, Umpierre SA, Villamarzo G, et al. Comparison of the endocervical brush and the endocervical curettage for the evaluation of the endocervical canal. P R Health Sci J 1995;14(3):195–7.
21. Martin-Hirsch PP, Paraskevaidis E, Bryant A, et al. Surgery for cervical intraepithelial neoplasia. Cochrane Database Syst Rev 2010;(6):CD001318.

22. Kyrgiou M, Koliopoulos G, Martin-Hirsch P, et al. Obstetric outcomes after conservative treatment for intraepithelial or early invasive cervical lesions: systematic review and meta-analysis. Lancet 2006;367(9509):489–98.
23. Werner CL, Lo JY, Heffernan T, et al. Loop electrosurgical excision procedure and risk of preterm birth. Obstet Gynecol 2010;115(3):605–8.
24. American College of Obstetricians and Gynecologists. ACOG Practice Bulletin No. 99: management of abnormal cervical cytology and histology. Obstet Gynecol 2008;112(6):1419–44.
25. Santesso N, Schunemann H, Blumenthal P, et al. World Health Organization guidelines: use of cryotherapy for cervical intraepithelial neoplasia. Int J Gynaecol Obstet 2012;118(2):97–102.
26. World Health Organization, Department of Reproductive Health and Research and Department of Chronic Diseases and Health Promotion. Comprehensive cervical cancer control: a guide to essential practice. 2006. p. 284. Available at: www.who.int/reproductivehealth/publications/cancers/9241547006. Accessed November 3, 2013.
27. Sauvaget C, Muwonge R, Sankaranarayanan R. Meta-analysis of the effectiveness of cryotherapy in the treatment of cervical intraepithelial neoplasia. Int J Gynaecol Obstet 2013;120(3):218–23.

APPENDIX A: COLPOSCOPY/LEEP ASSESSMENT

PATIENT IDENTIFICATION (Patient plate)	VCU Medical Center - Women's Health @ Nelson Cinic Richmond, Va. 23298 **Colposcopy/LEEP** Assessment/Treatment

Hx & Phy: Age: ____ Ht: _____ Wt: _______ B/P: _____/______ P: ____ LMP: _______ Allergies: __________

G___ P____ A____ HCG ( ) Pos ( ) Neg Smoking Hx: Contraception: ______________________

STD Hx: 1st Coitus: # of Partners Lifetime:

Referral PAP: ____________________ HR HPV:____________________ Prior ABNL : __________________

Prior Treatment for Dysplasia:____

Medical History/Medications:

COLPOSCOPY	( ) Adequate Colposcopy ( ) Inadequate Colposcopy
CODE: AV-Abnormal Vasc…. Pattern C- Columnar Epithelium CA- Condyloma Acuminatum E-True Erosion L-Leukoplakia (hyper) Keratosis M- Mosaic P- Punctation SCJ- Squamo-columnar Junction AWE-Acetowhite Epithelium X – Biopsy Site(s)	Reid's Colposcopic Index: Margin:_____ Color:_____ Vessels:_____ Iodine:_____ Total Index:_____
	Diagnostics: Chlamydia ( ) Gonorrhea ( ) Pap Smear ( ) Wet prep ( )
	Procedure: Bx ( ) ECC ( ) EndoBx ( ) Cryo ( ) LEEP ( )
	Pre-procedure diagnosis:
	Attending:
	Resident:
IMPRESSION:	Anesthesia:
	EBL: ( ) None ( ) Minimal Loss ( ) ___________ml
	Complications:
RECOMMENDATIONS:	
	( ) No specimens removed ( ) Other Biopsies
FOLLOW UP Pending Histology:	
	Patient condition @ d/c: ( ) Stable ( ) Other

❑ **Instruction sheet given for Self Care After Colposcopy ________ Nurse Initials**

❑ **Instruction sheet given for Self Care After LEEP / Cryo ___________ Nurse Initials**

Pain medication given per M.D. order @ _______ Nurses Signature______________

Vulvar Procedures

Biopsy, Bartholin Abscess Treatment, and Condyloma Treatment

Edward J. Mayeaux Jr, MD[a], Danielle Cooper, MD[b,*]

KEYWORDS

- Vulvar biopsy • Punch biopsy • Shave biopsy • Shave excision
- Bartholin fistulization • Marsupialization • Skin LEEP • CO_2 laser

KEY POINTS

- Several benign, premalignant, and malignant lesions may arise on the vulva, and multiple types of procedures may be used to diagnose and treat these conditions.
- Punch and shave biopsies may be used to diagnose most vulvar conditions, but lesions suspected of being melanomas may best be diagnosed with narrow-margin excisional biopsies.
- Bartholin gland cysts and abscesses may be treated with several different treatment modalities, the most common of which are fistulization and marsupialization.
- Genital warts may be treated with several medical and surgical modalities to relieve symptoms.

INTRODUCTION

A variety of skin lesions from benign to premalignant and malignant can present on the vulva, and examination and biopsy are often necessary to diagnose these conditions. The vulva is best examined using a good source of white light and a magnification device, which can be a simple hand-held magnifying lens or a sophisticated colposcope.[1] Biopsy is indicated for unidentified lesions, areas suspicious for malignancy, atypical pigmented lesions, suspicious ulcerations, or lesions that do not resolve after standard therapy. The vulvar examination sometimes can be aided by application of 3% to 5% acetic acid. Acetic acid has the same effect on the vulva as it does on the nonkeratinized cells of the cervix and vagina. However, because of the keratinized

Disclosure: The authors have no relationships with a commercial company that has a direct financial interest in the subject matter or materials discussed.

[a] Department of Family and Preventive Medicine, University of South Carolina School of Medicine, 3209 Colonial Drive, Columbia, SC 29203, USA; [b] Department of Obstetrics and Gynecology, Louisiana State University Health Sciences Center, 1501 Kings Highway, Shreveport, LA 71130, USA

* Corresponding author.

E-mail address: dbaker1@lsuhsc.edu

Obstet Gynecol Clin N Am 40 (2013) 759–772
http://dx.doi.org/10.1016/j.ogc.2013.08.009 obgyn.theclinics.com
0889-8545/13/$ – see front matter

nature of the more external vulvar tissue, it is important to soak gauze with acetic acid and allow it to sit on the area, allowing examination for at least 5 minutes to highlight areas of acetowhitening or hyperkeratosis.[1]

ANATOMY

The vulva encompasses an area between the genitocrural folds laterally, the mons pubis anteriorly, and the perianal area posteriorly. This area includes the mons pubis, the labia minora and majora, clitoris, vestibule, Skene glands and ducts, hymen, Bartholin glands and ducts, urethral meatus, and vestibulovaginal bulbs. Some vulvologists also include the anus and distal anal tract in this description because this area is also at risk for human papillomavirus (HPV) infection and transformation. The majority of the vulva is covered by keratinized hair-bearing skin; the exception is the vestibule, which is partially covered by a nonkeratinized surface without skin appendages, and is contiguous with the vagina. The presence of skin appendages may influence the type of treatments used for specified conditions and their relative success rates. The vestibule has numerous gland openings: Skene ducts, Bartholin glands and ducts, and minor vestibular glands. The vulva is subject to numerous epithelial diseases, and this article expands on 3 common issues for providers who encounter patients with vulvar problems.

VULVAR BIOPSY

Vulvar biopsy is performed to diagnose epithelial abnormalities. The biopsy may be performed using a Keyes punch instrument, blade, or scissors. The choice of tool is generally determined by provider preference and equipment availability. Punch biopsy is especially useful for flat or slightly raised lesions, and scissors or cervical biopsy forceps are good for raised or pedunculated lesions. Scalpels or skin blades may be used to perform shave biopsies and/or excisions for any type of lesion.

Epithelial punch biopsy obtains a full-thickness skin specimen for diagnostic assessment. The technique has the advantages of being rapid and simple, and generally results in an acceptable final cosmetic appearance. Vulvar biopsy is typically performed using a 3- to 6-mm punch (Keyes punch). With small lesions, a punch that is slightly larger than the lesion can remove the entire visible lesion with the biopsy.[2] The diagnostic yield may be increased if the most suspicious or abnormal-appearing area (darkest, most raised, or most irregular contour) is biopsied. The exception to this is sclerotic or ulcerative lesions whereby the edge of the lesion, including a small amount of normal skin, should be sampled.[1,2]

Indications for vulvar biopsy

- Evaluation of lesions of uncertain origin
- Confirmation/exclusion of the presence of dysplasia or malignancy, including melanoma
- Evaluation of skin tumors such as basal cell carcinoma or Kaposi sarcoma
- Diagnosis of bullous skin disorders such as pemphigus vulgaris
- Diagnosis of inflammatory skin disorders such as discoid lupus
- Removal of small skin lesions such as intradermal nevi
- Diagnosis of atypical-appearing lesions
- Evaluation of lesions that do not response to therapy as expected

To perform a punch biopsy, prepare the area with povidone-iodine or chlorhexidine. Lidocaine solution (1%–2%) with epinephrine can be used to anesthetize the area of biopsy, although epinephrine should not be used in the clitoral region. A tuberculin syringe with a 30-gauge needle is appropriate for this area; however, particularly sensitive areas may require the additional use of a topical anesthetic. If the topical anesthetic creams are applied on a mucous membrane, anesthesia occurs much more quickly than the typical 30 to 60 minutes' recommended time for application on keratinized skin; however, this is an off-label use of the products. Inject local anesthetic into the dermis to raise a bleb in the skin (**Fig. 1**) under the lesion and beyond its edges.[3]

A circular defect is not easily closed, but an oval or ellipse may be created by stretching the skin perpendicular to the lines of least skin tension with the nondominant hand during the procedure (**Fig. 2**). Rotate the punch biopsy instrument with mild downward force around its center axis in a clockwise and counterclockwise back-and-forth motion until it traverses the full thickness of the skin. After the punch biopsy is performed, relax the nondominant hand; the circular defect becomes more oval, allowing for easier closure.[2] Stop the downward pressure as soon as the instrument completely penetrates the subcutaneous fat (**Fig. 3**). Do not insert the instrument to the hub in thin-skinned areas because this can damage underlying structures. However, if the blade does not transect the dermis completely around the circle, the specimen may be transected through the dermis, potentially producing a specimen with inadequate depth of biopsy. In this instance, place the blade in exactly the same cut and extend it deeper. Gently lift the specimen with a needle or pick-ups and then cut it free at the base (beneath the dermis) using scissors if necessary.

After the biopsy, apply moderate pressure and, possibly, a hemostatic agent to stem bleeding, such as aluminum chloride, silver nitrate, or Monsel solution. Keep in mind that the latter 2 agents may cause tissue tattooing.[3] Monsel solution may produce tissue artifacts that can be troublesome to the pathologist if rebiopsy or further excision of a lesion becomes necessary.[4] Electrocautery can also be used to stop bleeding. Consider closing the biopsy site with a cyanoacrylate tissue adhesive, Steri-Strips, or an interrupted suture (**Fig. 4**), especially with larger biopsies (>4 mm), to decrease postprocedure pain and improve cosmesis. Suturing with absorbable sutures may eliminate the need for removal, but stiff sutures often irritate the vulva, making silk sutures preferable, especially on mucous membranes.

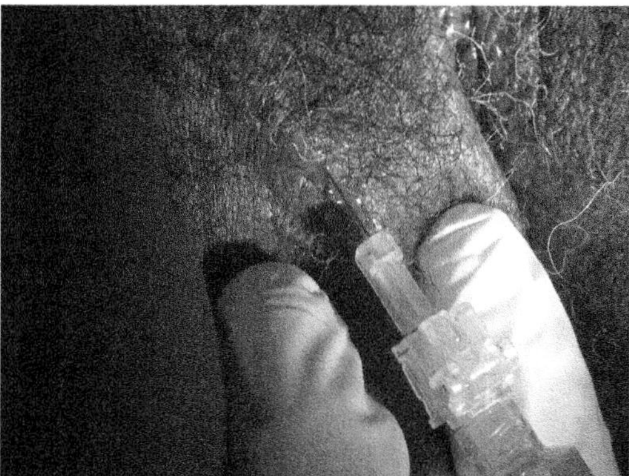

Fig. 1. To anesthetize the skin for a punch biopsy, inject lidocaine solution (1%–2%) with epinephrine into the dermis to raise a bleb in the skin under the lesion and beyond its edges.

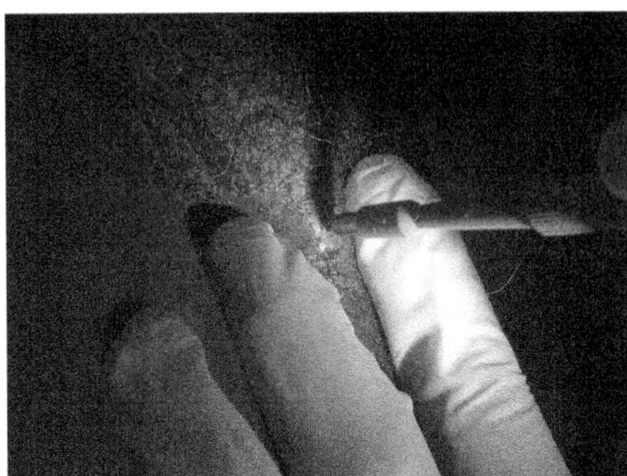

Fig. 2. Create an oval or elliptical defect by stretching the skin perpendicular to the lines of least skin tension with the nondominant hand during the procedure.

Pigmented lesions present a special problem because they may represent vulvar intraepithelial neoplasia (VIN), squamous cell carcinoma (SCC), or melanoma. One potential issue with punch or incisional biopsy that is raised historically is whether establishing a defect in the middle of a tumor allows for seeding or spread of the tumor. This theory has largely been disproven and is not considered clinically relevant.[5–7] Clinical examination is widely used for evaluation of melanoma risk in pigmented lesions. The ABCDE rule (Asymmetry, Border, Color, Diameter, and Evolution) is commonly used to assess risk.[8] Evolution is especially important in patients who are elderly, as a changing lesion in an elderly patient is more likely to be melanoma.[9] Biopsy also is recommended for a lesion that is distinct from other lesions on the patient's body ("ugly duckling" sign).[10] The American Academy of Dermatology (AAD) has recently issued a position statement on the management of melanomas. The AAD recommends a narrow excisional biopsy with 1- to 3-mm margins to clear the subclinical component in pigmented lesions considered at risk for melanoma. This biopsy can be accomplished in several ways, including elliptical excision with sutures or a deep shave removal to a depth below the anticipated plane of the lesion. If the suspicion for melanoma is high, most melanoma experts recommend performing deep shave (saucerization biopsy) or excisional biopsy so as to have the entire lesion available for evaluation.[11]

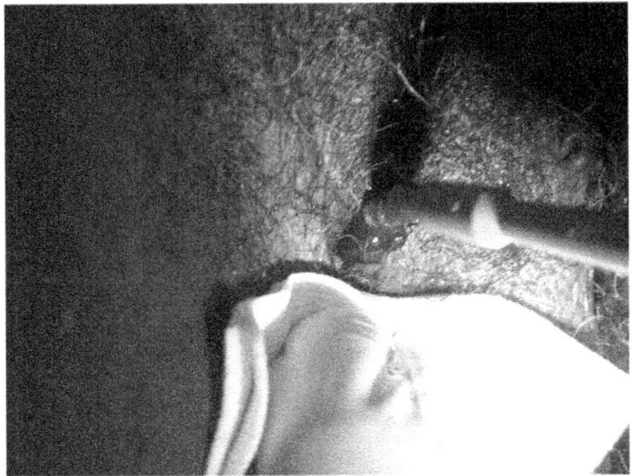

Fig. 3. Stop the downward pressure and remove the instrument as soon as the instrument completely penetrates the subcutaneous fat.

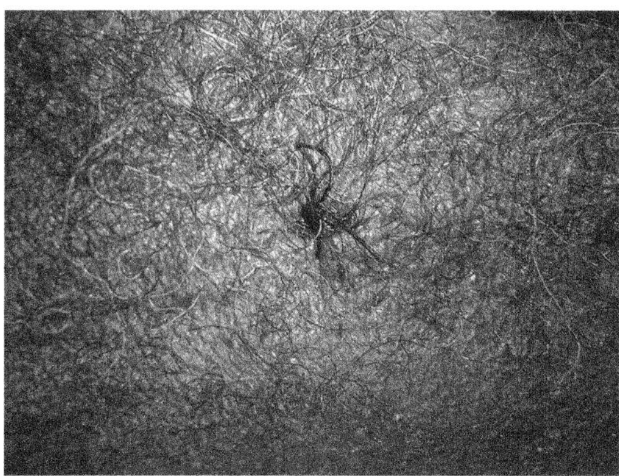

Fig. 4. Consider closing the biopsy site with an interrupted suture, especially with larger biopsies (>4 mm), to decrease the postprocedure pain and improve cosmesis. Stiff sutures often irritate the vulva, making silk sutures preferable, especially on mucous membranes.

To perform a shave biopsy, inject local anesthetic into the dermis under the lesion and beyond its edges. The wheal created expands the dermis, making the lesion easier to shave to an appropriate depth without penetrating to the fat layer, which makes scarring more likely. Squeeze skin between the thumb and forefinger of the nondominant hand to further elevate the lesion. For macular or raised nonsuspicious lesions, a simple shave biopsy is appropriate. Hold a blade parallel to the skin and shallowly remove a thin disk below the level of pigmentation. In a saucerization biopsy, a thick disk of tissue is removed with a scalpel, Dermablade, or curved razor blade, yielding a specimen that extends to at least the mid-dermis (1–4 mm deep).[3,12] Hold the blade at a 45° angle to the skin, bend or bow the blade (depending on the width of lesion) to achieve adequate depth of cut, and remove a disk of tissue deep into the dermis with 1 to 2 mm of surrounding normal skin laterally.[12] The base of the shave should be in the dermis with multiple bleeding points before hemostasis, have no subcutaneous fat apparent, and not have any apparent lesion remaining (**Fig. 5**). If an area of pigment remains after saucerization, perform a punch or excisional biopsy and submit both specimens in the same pathology container. Use a hemostatic agent or electrocautery for hemostasis. Dress the site with an ointment. Instruct the patient to keep the area moist with ointment or petrolatum and to keep covered for at least 1 week.[3]

BARTHOLIN CYST/ABSCESS

The Bartholin glands (greater vestibular glands) are a pair of pea-sized mucus-secreting vestibular glands located at the 5 o'clock and 7 o'clock positions at the vaginal introitus. These glands are normally not palpable or visible. Cysts of these glands develop because of blockage of the duct, often caused by infection or trauma. Symptomatic Bartholin abscesses and cysts account for about 2% of all gynecologic visits per year.[13] The affected patient typically reports vulvar pain, dyspareunia, and/or pain with walking or sitting. If the cyst develops into an abscess, the symptoms tend to be severe or even incapacitating. In addition to local symptoms, the patient may report subjective fevers, nausea, and influenza-like symptoms.

There are many treatment options for symptomatic Bartholin cysts or abscesses, including simple drainage, fistulization, marsupialization, and excision of the gland.[14] Destruction of the cyst or abscess base after drainage with silver nitrate or alcohol

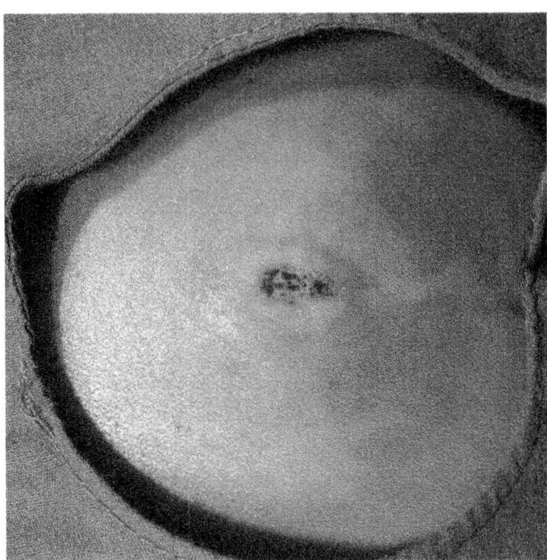

Fig. 5. After a shave, the base should be in the dermis with multiple bleeding points before hemostasis, have no subcutaneous fat apparent, and not have any apparent lesion remaining.

has been reported. The carbon dioxide (CO_2) laser may be used to ablate fenestration or excise the gland. If a patient's Bartholin gland cyst ruptures spontaneously, only hot sitz baths during resolution are needed.[15] Antibiotics are only necessary when secondary infection develops or sexually transmitted infections are identified.[15] Regardless of the method used, the provider and any assistants should take personal-protection precautions and wear gloves and eye equipment during these procedures.

Simple incision and drainage of the abscess under local anesthesia will provide prompt symptom relief, but reoccurrence after this procedure is common.[15] Following a 1- to 2-cm incision in the cyst, the wall may be ablated with a stick of crystalloid silver nitrate inserted into the cavity. The coagulum may be removed or allowed to spontaneously drain.[16,17] The most common adverse effects are vulvar burning on postoperative day1 and labial edema. Healing usually occurs within 10 days.[14] Hemorrhage is reported in 4% to 5% of these patients.[18,19] Simple needle aspiration, sometimes with ethyl chloride spray for anesthesia, has also been studied.[20–23] However, compared with alcohol sclerotherapy, needle aspiration has been associated with more than twice the frequency of recurrence, with no statistical analysis reported.[20] Needle aspiration and irrigation with 70% alcohol for 5 minutes followed by reevacuation has been studied.[20] Transient hyperemia and hematoma has been reported in many patients.[20] Seventeen percent of patients in one study experienced tissue necrosis and scarring, so the method is not widely used.[24]

Bartholin cyst or abscess fistulization involves creating a new, epithelialized outflow tract for an obstructed Bartholin lesion by placing a Word catheter (Rusch Corp, Duluth, GA), a 14F Foley catheter, or a Jacobi ring.[25–27] Prep the area with povidone-iodine or chlorhexidine. Local anesthesia is achieved by injecting the area around and under the lesion (**Fig. 6**) with lidocaine with epinephrine. This field block may take up to 10 minutes to work. Be careful not to inject the anesthetic into the cyst or abscess itself, as this often produces inadequate anesthesia and may result in explosive decompression of the lesion when incised. Next, insert a Word catheter through a 3- to 5-mm stab incision on the inner labium minus (just external to the

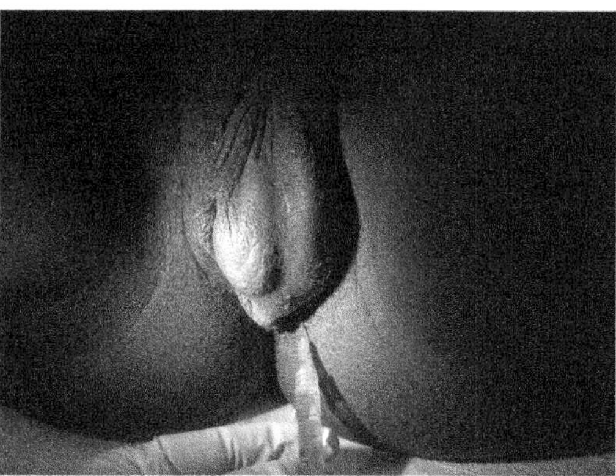

Fig. 6. Local anesthesia for a Bartholin cyst or abscess fistulization is achieved by injecting the area around and under the lesion with lidocaine with epinephrine. This field block may take up to 10 minutes to work.

hymenal ring) into the Bartholin gland lesion (**Fig. 7**). Hemostats or a probe should be used to break up any loculations present. The bulb of the catheter is inflated (**Fig. 8**) with 3 mL of sterile saline or gel (not air), and the catheter is tucked into the vagina and left in place for up to 4 weeks.[28]

The Jacobi ring is made from an 8F flexible catheter threaded over a 2-0 silk suture, fashioned into a ring that enters and leaves the cyst or abscess through 2 separate incisions.[27] Recurrent Bartholin-gland pathology is noted in 4% to 17% of patients after fistulization.[14] In a randomized trial comparing the Word catheter with the Jacobi ring for symptomatic Bartholin duct abscesses, healing was accomplished by 3 weeks and patients were highly satisfied in both groups.[29]

Marsupialization (window operation) of the cyst or abscess is another treatment option and is often preferred if the patient has previously failed Word catheter placement. This procedure involves excising an elliptical portion of vestibular skin and cyst wall, breaking up any loculations within the cyst and suturing the cyst-wall edges with interrupted absorbable 3-0 suture to the surrounding vestibular and introital tissue.[28] For

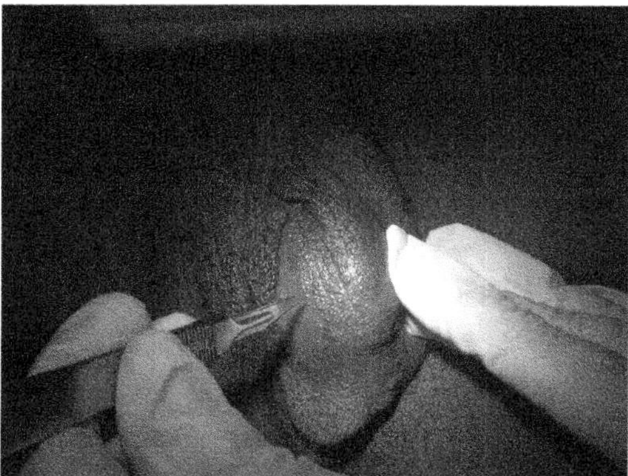

Fig. 7. A Word catheter is inserted through a 3- to 5-mm stab incision on the inner labium minus (just external to the hymenal ring) into the Bartholin gland lesion, and inflated with saline or gel.

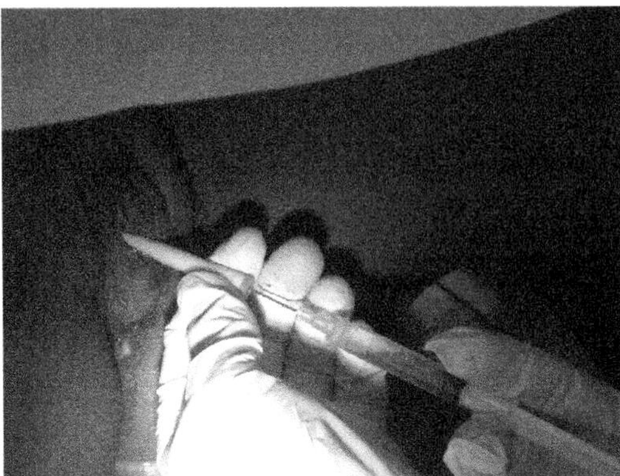

Fig. 8. The bulb of the catheter is inflated through the stem with 3 mL of sterile saline or gel, as air may prematurely deflate the catheter.

best results, it is ideal to perform this procedure on uninfected tissue. Typically this procedure is performed in an outpatient surgical suite, although it is possible in an office setting if the patient can tolerate the local/regional anesthetic for the procedure.[14] Median healing occurred in less than 2 weeks but with bleeding being reported in 11% of patients in one study.[30] Recurrence after marsupialization is 10% to 15%. Keep in mind that if the cyst develops in a postmenopausal patient, a biopsy should be taken from the cyst wall to be evaluated by the pathologist for malignancy.[31]

The CO_2 laser may be used under local anesthesia to create an opening in the vulvar skin in the area of the duct orifice, and the lesion contents evacuated.[32–35] The remaining wall may be left intact, ablated, or excised.[32] Healing generally occurs in an average of 2.2 weeks. Unfortunately, reported recurrences are common,[30,36] and sometimes prolonged healing may interfere with daily activities and intercourse.[14] Major bleeding occurs in 2% to 8% of patients after laser ablation.[33,34] Bartholin gland excision can be considered in cases of recurrence or suspected malignancy. Bleeding or hematoma was reported in 2% to 8%, fever in 24%, and persistent dyspareunia in 8% to 16% of patients.[32,37,38]

TREATMENT OF VULVAR CONDYLOMA

Genital warts (condyloma acuminata) affect approximately 1% of the population.[39] Low-oncogenic-risk HPV viral types 6 and 11 cause more than 90% of anogenital warts. More than two-thirds of individuals infected with HPV have a transient infection that is subsequently cleared by the host immune response.[40] The average HPV infection in adolescent females lasts a median of 5.6 months.[41] Diagnosis of genital warts is usually made by visual inspection.[42] A biopsy should be taken of any lesion that has an atypical appearance, is pigmented, or is resistant to therapy.[43] The quadrivalent HPV vaccine can prevent infection with HPV-6 and HPV-11, but does not treat existing lesions.[44]

The primary goal of the treatment of vulvar condyloma is to remove symptomatic warts. Because many warts will regress over time, treatments that do not have a significant risk of scarring should be considered first. All treatment modalities have high recurrence rates and variable success rates. No definitive evidence suggests that any of the available treatments are superior to any other, and no single treatment is ideal for all patients or all warts. Practitioners should be familiar with at least 1 patient-applied treatment (eg, imiquimod, podofilox, or sinecatechins) and 1 provider-applied therapy (eg, surgical excision, cryotherapy, trichloroacetic acid [TCA]).[43] Choosing an appropriate treatment modality for condyloma depends on the size, number, and location of the lesions, as well as provider training. The use of tailored therapies to the specific needs and situation of the patient can produce good outcomes for the majority.

Imiquimod cream (Aldara and Zyclara; Medicis Pharmaceuticals, Scottsdale, AZ) is indicated only for external HPV infections (**Table 1**), and is contraindicated for use on occluded mucous membranes or on the cervix.[42] The cream should be rubbed into the lesion to promote absorption. Patients are advised to wash the affected area with soap and water 6 to 10 hours after application.[45] Side effects include erythema, erosion, itching, skin flaking, and edema. In 3 randomized placebo-controlled trials of 5% cream, 37% to 54% of treated patients showed clearance within 16 weeks.[46]

A biologically active extract of podophyllin, podofilox (Condylox; Watson Pharma, San Antonio, TX) 0.5% gel, solution, or cream, is indicated for patient application to genital lesions (see **Table 1**). It is contraindicated for use in the vagina, urethra, perianal area, cervix, and in pregnancy. There have been reported deaths from application of podophyllin to occluded membranes, so this type of use is strictly contraindicated.[43] Follow-up is usually within 4 weeks, and thereafter until healing. Placebo-controlled trials have shown 45% to 77% clearance rates within 4 to 6 weeks. Side effects include local inflammation, irritation, erosion, burning, pain, and itching.[46]

Sinecatechins ointment, a green-tea extract, may be used for external warts.[47–49] The medication should not be washed off after use. The most common side effects of sinecatechins are erythema, pruritus/burning, pain, ulceration, edema, induration, and vesicular rash. It also may weaken condoms and diaphragms. The safety and efficacy of the medication is not established for persons infected by human immunodeficiency virus, immunocompromised persons, persons with clinical genital herpes, or pregnant females.

Provider-administered therapies to treat genital warts involve excisions, ablations, and application of topical agents. Excisional procedures may be done in an outpatient setting for milder disease, or in an operating-room setting for more extensive disease. Provider administration has the advantage of eliminating most or all warts at a single visit. Vulvar condyloma must be resected down to normal skin, after which the base is cauterized. A #15 blade or scissors can be used to resect the condyloma using a shave technique as described earlier, after which a cautery tool or chemical applied to the area is used to control bleeding. Suture is usually unnecessary.

The skin loop electrosurgical excisional procedure (LEEP) is an excellent modality for the treatment of perineal condylomata in both males and females, and the basic equipment needed is already present in many providers' offices. HPV DNA has been found in laser and electrocoagulation smoke, although it is not known if viable HPV is present.[50] Theoretically HPV could also be present in LEEP smoke, so operators should wear a virus-filtering mask when removing condyloma in this fashion.[51] Loops for the removal of external lesions are typically smaller and shorter than standard cervical loops, and are selected to allow easy removal of the lesion. The loops for the removal of condyloma typically are smaller and shorter than the typical cervical loop, allowing for easier control with resection. Local anesthesia is injected intradermally. The loop is introduced into normal skin near the base of the lesion and is pulled completely under the lesion through the dermis. Any remaining lesion is then carefully

Table 1
Therapies for condyloma acuminata

Drug	Applied by	Pregnancy	Treatment Areas	Notes
Imiquimod 5% cream	Patient	No	Vulva	Apply to lesions 3 times a week, every other day, for up to 16 wk. Wash with soap and water after 6–10 h
Podofilox 0.5% solution or gel	Patient	No	Vulva	Apply to lesions twice daily for 3 d, then 4 consecutive days of no therapy each week for a maximum of 4 wk
Sinecatechins 15% ointment	Patient	No	Vulva	Apply a 0.5-cm strand to each wart 3 times daily using a finger to ensure coverage with a thin layer of ointment for up to 16 wk
Cryotherapy with liquid nitrogen	Provider	Yes	Vulva, vagina, anal	Refrigerant is applied until an ice-ball forms for 2–3 mm beyond the lesion margin
Cryotherapy with a nitrous oxide or carbon dioxide cryoprobe	—	—	Vulva	Refrigerant is applied until an ice-ball forms 2–3 mm beyond the lesion margin
Podophyllin	Provider	No	Vulva	Apply to each wart and allow to air-dry to prevent spread to adjacent areas
Trichloroacetic acid 50%–90% solution	Provider	Yes	Vulva, vagina, anal	Apply a small amount only to the warts and allow to dry
Surgical removal (sharp, electrocautery, curettage)	—	Yes	Vulva, anal	—
Laser	—	Yes	Vulva, vagina	—

Data from Workowski KA, Berman S, Centers for Disease Control and Prevention (CDC). Sexually transmitted diseases treatment guidelines, 2010. MMWR Recomm Rep 2010;59(RR-12):1–110; and Mayeaux EJ Jr, Dunton C. Modern management of external genital warts. J Low Genit Tract Dis 2008;12:185–92.

shaved down to the dermis using the side of the loop and fine paint-brush style cuts (**Fig. 9**). Fulguration can be used for hemostasis, but is not usually necessary. Late bleeding has been reported in 4% of patients treated for vaginal lesions, and can usually be controlled with Monsel solution or fulguration. Infection is an uncommon complication. Hypopigmentation and hypertrophic scars are rarely reported.[43]

Podophyllin resin (10%–25%) may be applied weekly.[42] Application should be limited to less than 0.5 mL of podophyllin per session, and the treatment area should not contain any open lesions or wounds, to prevent absorption of the toxin. The

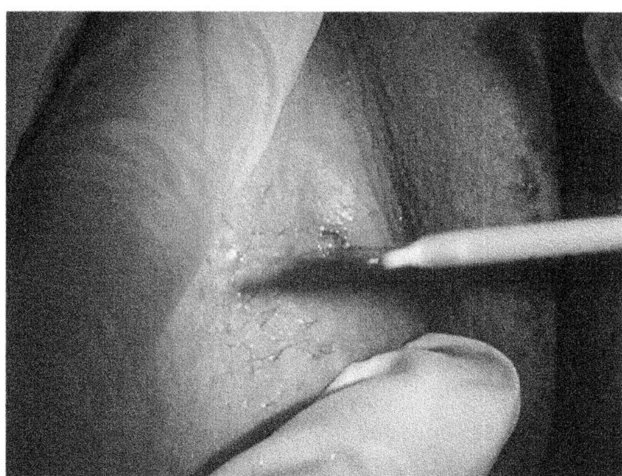

Fig. 9. During an electrosurgical shave, the loop is introduced into normal skin near the base of the lesion and pulled completely under the lesion through the dermis. Any remaining lesion is then carefully shaved down to the dermis using the side of the loop and fine paint-brush style cuts. Note that a cervical loop is used here for visualization, but shorter skin loops are easier to use.

preparation should be thoroughly washed off 1 to 4 hours after application to reduce local irritation. Podophyllin resin preparations differ in the concentration of active components and contaminants.

The CO_2 laser can be used to excise the base of a pedunculated lesion or desiccate a flat lesion just beyond the dermal layer. Appropriate personal-protective equipment including safety goggles are a necessity. Providers must remember to place moist gauze in the rectum to prevent possible ignition of colonic gas. With this procedure, healing occurs by secondary intention; there is rarely bleeding to control because of the superficial nature of the procedure. The importance of pain control and healing techniques are stressed to the patient. Sitz baths 3 times a day and lidocaine ointments for pain control will typically be adequate. HPV DNA has been found in the "plume of smoke" associated with the laser; therefore, a virus-filtering mask must be worn and a smoke evacuator used to minimize possible exposure.[51]

Cryotherapy is a commonly used method to remove warts, and is likely the safest modality during pregnancy. Freezing with liquid nitrogen may involve some pain and bleeding. Liquid nitrogen should be applied via a spray device or cotton-tipped applicator, or nitrous oxide or CO_2 via a cryoprobe, until an ice-ball forms 2 to 3 mm beyond the margin of the lesion. Local anesthesia can be used, although many patients will tolerate the cryotherapy without any such treatment. After several days the treated tissue will slough off; inflammation ensues and then subsides as healing occurs.[42]

TCA is used to treat external condyloma but is not recommended for use in the vagina, cervix, or urinary meatus. TCA can be prepared in different strengths and must be compounded at a pharmacy. A thin cotton-tip applicator is used to apply the acid directly to the lesion until a white frost develops. If pain is intense, the acid can be neutralized with soap or sodium bicarbonate. Excess liquid can ulcerate surrounding tissue, and petroleum jelly can be applied to protect unaffected skin. Multiple weekly applications may be required to adequately treat the condyloma.[42]

In general, genital warts will resolve with therapy within 1 to 6 months, regardless of the choice of treatment. Patients need to be aware of the nature of the HPV disease and the potential for latency and viral reactivation. Condom use should be encouraged, although at this time prevention is only possible with vaccination.

REFERENCES

1. Haefner H, Mayeaux EJ Jr. Vulvar abnormalities. In: Mayeaux EJ Jr, Cox T, editors. Modern colposcopy. 3rd edition. Philadelphia: Lippincott, Williams, Wilkins; 2011. p. 432–70.
2. Mayeaux EJ Jr. Punch biopsy of the skin. In: Mayeaux EJ Jr, editor. The essential guide to primary care procedures. Philadelphia: Wolters Kluwer: Lippincott, Williams, Wilkins; 2009. p. 187–94.
3. Pickett H. Shave and punch biopsy for skin lesions. Am Fam Physician 2011; 84(9):995–1002.
4. Olmstead PM, Lund HZ, Leonard DD. Monsel's solution: a histologic nuisance. J Am Acad Dermatol 1980;3(5):492–8.
5. Pflugfelder A, Weide B, Eigentler TK, et al. Incisional biopsy and melanoma prognosis: facts and controversies. Clin Dermatol 2010;28(3):316–8.
6. Sober AJ, Balch CM. Method of biopsy and incidence of positive margins in primary melanoma. Ann Surg Oncol 2007;14(2):274–5.
7. Lin SW, Kaye V, Goldfarb N, et al. Melanoma tumor seeding after punch biopsy. Dermatol Surg 2012;38(7 Pt 1):1083–5.
8. Thomas L, Tranchand P, Berard F, et al. Semiological value of ABCDE criteria in the diagnosis of cutaneous pigmented tumors. Dermatology 1998;197: 11–7.
9. Banky JP, Kelly JW, English DR, et al. Incidence of new and changed nevi and melanomas detected using baseline images and dermoscopy in patients at high risk for melanoma. Arch Dermatol 2005;141:998–1006.
10. Grob JJ, Bonerandi JJ. The 'ugly duckling' sign: identification of the common characteristics of nevi in an individual as a basis for melanoma screening. Arch Dermatol 1998;134:103–4.
11. Bichakjian CK, Halpern AC, Johnson TM, et al. Guidelines of care for the management of primary cutaneous melanoma. J Am Acad Dermatol 2011;65(5): 1032–47.
12. Tran KT, Wright NA, Cockerell CJ. Biopsy of the pigmented lesion—when and how. J Am Acad Dermatol 2008;59(5):852–71.
13. Pundir J, Auld BJ. A review of the management of diseases of the Bartholin's gland. J Obstet Gynaecol 2008;28(2):161–5.
14. Wechter ME, Wu JM, Marzano D, et al. Management of Bartholin duct cysts and abscesses: a systematic review. Obstet Gynecol Surv 2009;64(6): 395–404.
15. Omole F, Simmons BJ, Hacker Y. Management of Bartholin's duct cyst and gland abscess. Am Fam Physician 2003;68(1):135–40.
16. Ergeneli MH. Silver nitrate for Bartholin gland cysts. Eur J Obstet Gynecol Reprod Biol 1999;82:231–2.
17. Ozdegirmenci O, Kayikcioglu F, Haberal A. Prospective randomized study of marsupialization versus silver nitrate application in the management of Bartholin gland cysts and abscesses. J Minim Invasive Gynecol 2009;16(2): 149–52.
18. Ortac UF, Dunder I, Alatas C, et al. Management of Bartholin's cysts and abscesses with silver nitrate ($AgNO_3$). Turk J Med Sci 1991;15:116–24.
19. Turan C, Vicdan K, Gokmen O. The treatment of Bartholin's cyst and abscess with silver nitrate. Int J Gynaecol Obstet 1995;48:317–8.
20. Cobellis PL, Stradella L, De Lucia E, et al. Alcohol sclerotherapy: a new method for Bartholin gland cyst treatment. Minerva Ginecol 2006;58:245–8.

21. Cheetham DR. Bartholin's cyst: marsupialization or aspiration? Am J Obstet Gynecol 1985;152:569–70.
22. Poma PA. Bartholin's duct abscess: office management. Proc Inst Med Chic 1982;35:85–6.
23. van Bogaert LJ. Management of Bartholin's abscess. World Health Forum 1997; 18:200–1.
24. Kafali H, Yurtseven S, Ozardali I. Aspiration and alcohol sclerotherapy: a novel method for management of Bartholin's cyst or abscess. Eur J Obstet Gynecol Reprod Biol 2004;112:98–101.
25. Haider Z, Condous G, Kirk E, et al. The simple outpatient management of Bartholin's abscess using the Word catheter: a preliminary study. Aust N Z J Obstet Gynaecol 2007;47:137–40.
26. Yavetz H, Lessing JB, Jaffa AJ, et al. Fistulization: an effective treatment for Bartholin's abscesses and cysts. Acta Obstet Gynecol Scand 1987;66:63–4.
27. Gennis P, Li SF, Provataris J, et al. Jacobi ring catheter treatment of Bartholin's abscesses. Am J Emerg Med 2005;23:414–5.
28. Mayeaux EJ Jr. Bartholin's gland cysts and abscesses treatment. In: Mayeaux EJ Jr, editor. The essential guide to primary care procedures. Philadelphia: Wolters Kluwer: Lippincott, Williams, Wilkins; 2009. p. 497–503.
29. Gennis P, Li SF, Provataris J, et al. Randomized pilot study comparing a rubber ring catheter to the word catheter in the treatment of Bartholin abscesses. Acad Emerg Med 2004;11:527.
30. Downs MC, Randall HW Jr. The ambulatory surgical management of Bartholin duct cysts. J Emerg Med 1989;7:623–6.
31. Schorge JO, Schaffer JI, Halvorson LM, et al. Williams gynecology. 2008:675.
32. Penna C, Fambrini M, Fallani MG. CO_2 laser treatment for Bartholin's gland cyst. Int J Gynaecol Obstet 2002;76:79–80.
33. Heinonen PK. Carbon dioxide laser in the treatment of abscess and cyst of Bartholin's gland. J Obstet Gynaecol 1990;10:535–7.
34. Fambrini M, Penna C, Pieralli A, et al. Carbon-dioxide laser vaporization of the Bartholin gland cyst: a retrospective analysis on 200 cases. J Minim Invasive Gynecol 2008;15:327–31.
35. Benedetti Panici P, Manci N, Bellati F, et al. CO_2 laser therapy of the Bartholin's gland cyst: surgical data and functional short- and long-term results. J Minim Invasive Gynecol 2007;14:348–51.
36. Goldberg JE. Simplified treatment for disease of Bartholin's gland. Obstet Gynecol 1970;35:109–10.
37. Mungan T, Ugur M, Yalcin H, et al. Treatment of Bartholin's cyst and abscess: excision versus silver nitrate insertion. Eur J Obstet Gynecol Reprod Biol 1995;63:61–3.
38. Rouzier R, Azarian M, Plantier F, et al. Unusual presentation of Bartholin's gland duct cysts: anterior expansions. BJOG 2005;112:1150–2.
39. Gunter J. Genital and perianal warts: new treatment opportunities for human papillomavirus infection. Am J Obstet Gynecol 2003;189(Suppl 3):S3–11.
40. Ho GY, Bierman R, Beardsley L, et al. Natural history of cervicovaginal papillomavirus infection in young women. N Engl J Med 1998;338:423–8.
41. Brown DR, Shew ML, Qadadri B, et al. A longitudinal AQ8 study of genital human papillomavirus infection in a cohort of closely followed adolescent women. J Infect Dis 2005;191:182–92.
42. Workowski KA, Berman S, Centers for Disease Control and Prevention (CDC). Sexually transmitted diseases treatment guidelines, 2010. MMWR Recomm Rep 2010;59(RR-12):1–110.

43. Mayeaux EJ Jr, Dunton C. Modern management of external genital warts. J Low Genit Tract Dis 2008;12:185–92.
44. FUTURE I/II Study Group, Dillner J, Kjaer SK. Four year efficacy of prophylactic human papillomavirus quadrivalent vaccine against low grade cervical, vulvar, and vaginal intraepithelial neoplasia and anogenital warts: randomised controlled trial. BMJ 2010;340:c3493.
45. Ferenczy A. Treatment of external genital warts. J Low Genit Tract Dis 2000;4: 128–34.
46. Wiley DJ, Douglas JM, Beutner K, et al. External genital warts: diagnosis, treatment and prevention. Clin Infect Dis 2002;35(Suppl 2):S210–24.
47. Tatti S, Swinehart JM, Thielert C, et al. Sinecatechins, a defined green tea extract, in the treatment of external anogenital warts: a randomized controlled trial. Obstet Gynecol 2008;111:1371–9.
48. Stockfleth E, Beti H, Orasan R, et al. Topical Polyphenon E in the treatment of external genital and perianal warts: a randomized controlled trial. Br J Dermatol 2008;158:1329–38.
49. Gross G, Meyer KG, Pres H, et al. A randomized, double-blind, four-arm parallel-group, placebo-controlled Phase II/III study to investigate the clinical efficacy of two galenic formulations of Polyphenon E in the treatment of external genital warts. J Eur Acad Dermatol Venereol 2007;21:1404–12.
50. Sawchuk WS, Weber PJ, Lowy DR, et al. Infectious papillomavirus in the vapor of warts treated with carbon dioxide laser or electrocoagulation: detection and protection. J Am Acad Dermatol 1989;21:41–9.
51. Mayeaux EJ, Harper MB, Barksdale W, et al. Noncervical human papillomavirus genital infections. Am Fam Physician 1995;52(4):1137–46.

Cystoscopy and Other Urogynecologic Procedures

Jonathan L. Gleason, MD

KEYWORDS

• Urogynecology • Cystoscopy • Office procedures

KEY POINTS

- Office-based procedures are increasingly available for diagnostic and therapeutic purposes in urogynecology.
- Cystourethroscopy can be safely performed in the office setting, and is often used for diagnostic purposes and treatment of lower urinary tract symptoms.
- The treatment of stress urinary incontinence, urge urinary incontinence, and surgical complications is sometimes feasible in the office.
- Appropriate patient selection is important in all office-based procedures.

CYSTOURETHROSCOPY

Indications/Contraindications

Cystourethroscopy is performed to visualize the urethra and the bladder. There are several diagnostic and therapeutic indications within the scope of female pelvic medicine and reconstructive surgery (FPMRS) (**Table 1**). The presence of a current urinary tract infection is a relative contraindication to cystourethroscopy because urinary tract instrumentation may exacerbate an infection.

Technique/Procedure

Rigid cystoscope

A rigid cystoscope comprises 3 components: the telescope, bridge, and sheath. Telescopes are available with several viewing angles. Zero-degree telescopes are useful for urethroscopy and periurethral bulking procedures. Thirty-degree telescopes are useful for obtaining biopsies and for intravesical injections. Seventy-degree telescopes are the most commonly used scopes for diagnostic purposes within the bladder.

The bridge is the connection between the telescope and the sheath, and may contain ports for introduction of instruments into the bladder. For office-based procedures, a single port should suffice.

Female Pelvic Medicine and Reconstructive Surgery, Carilion Clinic, Virginia Tech Carilion School of Medicine, 101 Elm Avenue, Suite 400, Roanoke, VA 24013, USA
E-mail address: jlgleason@carilionclinic.org

Obstet Gynecol Clin N Am 40 (2013) 773–785
http://dx.doi.org/10.1016/j.ogc.2013.09.003 **obgyn.theclinics.com**
0889-8545/13/$ – see front matter

Table 1
Indications and contraindications for cystourethroscopy in the office

Indications		
Diagnostic	**Therapeutic**	**Contraindications[a]**
Hematuria: gross or persistent microscopic	Removal of foreign body	Urinary tract infection
Lower urinary tract symptoms	Intravesical onabotulinumtoxinA injection	Relative contraindication: history of autonomic dysreflexia[a]
Refractory urinary incontinence	Periurethral bulking agent injection	—
Recurrent urinary tract infections	—	—
Evaluation of surgical complications: suspected foreign body	—	—
Evaluation of urogenital fistulas and urethral diverticula	—	—
Sudden and recent onset of lower urinary tract symptoms	—	—
Incongruence of urodynamic findings and patient symptoms	—	—
Persistent or severe bladder pain	—	—

[a] Spinal cord patients with injury level above T6 may develop sudden-onset malignant hypertension.

The sheath covers the telescope and contains the inflow and outflow for distention media. The 17F sheath is the smallest, and is the one most commonly used for diagnostic cystoscopy. Larger sheaths are necessary for introduction of instrumentation, but may cause more discomfort.

Flexible cystoscope

The flexible cystoscope combines the sheath and the telescope components of the rigid cystoscope. The tip of a flexible scope ranges from 15F to 18F. Flexible scopes are more fragile, and must be handled with care. Furthermore, flexible scopes have a lower flow rate because of the smaller-caliber lumen. There is no evidence that flexible cystoscopes are less morbid or better tolerated in women.[1]

Distending media

The most commonly used distending media are water, saline, and glycine. Water is ideal for diagnostic cystoscopy because of its cost and availability. Saline must be used when performing prolonged procedures whereby absorption into the vascular space is a consideration, but this is unlikely to be a concern in office-based procedures. Glycine is commonly used if electrocautery is being performed, and should be considered any time a biopsy is being obtained. The distending media should be placed 80 to 100 cm above the patient's pubic symphysis.

Technique

Diagnostic

The urethral meatus is cleaned with disinfectant and the urethra is prepared using sterile, water-soluble lubricant. There is no evidence that intraurethral lidocaine reduces discomfort in women undergoing cystourethroscopy.[2] The cystoscope is then inserted with the distending media running with or without the use of an obturator. The bladder should be surveyed in its entirety in a stepwise fashion to visualize all 4 quadrants of the bladder, the ureteral orifices, and the trigone. Urethroscopy can be performed during withdrawal, and is facilitated by using either a 30° or 0° telescope.

Operative

Common office procedures include bladder biopsy and intravesical injection of onabotulinumtoxinA for refractory overactive bladder. The use of operative cystourethroscopy is limited in the office setting, owing to patient intolerance of a larger sheath and a longer procedure.

Bladder biopsy is performed by inserting a biopsy forceps through the operative port on the bridge of a rigid cystoscope. A small sample of the tissue is removed. If bleeding is encountered, an electrocautery device is used sparingly to control bleeding.

Injection of onabotulinumtoxinA into the bladder is a straightforward technique. Thirty minutes before the procedure, the bladder is instilled with 30 mL of 2% lidocaine. OnabotulinumtoxinA is a powder that is fixed to the walls of the bottle in which it is presented. Ten milliliters of injectable saline is slowly introduced into the bottle containing the medication, and the bottle is then gently swirled to bring the onabotulinumtoxinA into solution. Care should be taken to avoid rigorous introduction of the saline and shaking of the bottle, because this produces bubbles in the bottle and makes it difficult to withdraw the medication. The medication is then withdrawn from the bottle into a sterile syringe, which is then attached to the long needle that will pass through the operative port of a cystoscope. The needle is flushed such that the medication is visible at the tip of the needle. Various methods have been described for injection, and typically involve injection of 0.5 mL of 10 units/mL solution per injection site starting just above the trigone in the bladder base, with rows running parallel to the interureteric ridge.[3] The author's routine practice is to perform 2 parallel rows of 7 injections, and 1 row of 6 injections.

Complications and Management

The most common complication of diagnostic cystourethroscopy is urinary tract infection, which occurs after 2% to 8% of cases.[4,5] This complication may be avoided by select use of prophylactic antibiotics in women at risk for developing urinary tract infections. Bleeding can occur during operative cystourethroscopy, and may be controlled with sparing use of electrocautery. It is imperative that the distending media be nonconducting (glycine) when using electrocautery. Risk factors for developing urinary tract infections after cystoscopy are listed in **Box 1**.

Box 1
Risk factors for developing urinary tract infections after cystoscopy

Advanced age

Anatomic anomalies of the urinary tract

Poor nutritional status

Smoking

Immunodeficiency including chronic steroid use

Data from Cruse PJ. Surgical wound infection. In: Wonsiewicz MJ, editor. Infectious disease. Philadelphia: WB Saunders; 1992. p. 758–64.

Postoperative Care

Routine use of antimicrobial prophylaxis is not recommended.[4,6] The authors suggest select use of antibiotics for patients with risk factors. In such cases, antibiotics are administered before the procedure and should be continued for 24 hours. Fluoroquinolones and trimethoprim-sulfamethoxazole are commonly used. Postoperative discomfort may be managed with nonsteroidal anti-inflammatory medications, taking a warm bath, holding a warm and damp washcloth over the urethra, and use of phenazopyridine for dysuria and bladder pain.

Reporting, Follow-Up, and Clinical Implications

Findings of the cystourethroscopy should be shared directly with the patient, and this may take place during the procedure to decrease patient anxiety. It is the author's practice to document a separate procedure note. Most diagnostic cystourethroscopy will have normal findings, allowing the patient and physician to move forward with the treatment of idiopathic conditions such as overactive bladder and dysuria, and providing reassurance that patients with lower urinary symptoms do not have a reparable anatomic finding, or malignancy, within the bladder. When evaluating a patient with a fistula or a complication from a prior pelvic reconstructive surgery, the location of the bladder anomaly may be useful for surgical planning.

Outcomes

Cystourethroscopy is the only means of direct visualization of the lower urinary tract.

Current Controversies

The role of cystourethroscopy in the evaluation of persistent or complex urinary incontinence is unclear. The evidence does not support the routine use of cystourethroscopy for evaluation of patients with simple urinary incontinence.[7] Practice patterns of the utilization of outpatient cystourethroscopy in the evaluation of refractory incontinence vary considerably. The primary role is to screen for bladder cancer, or abnormalities within the bladder, in women with persistent lower urinary tract symptoms, or in women at high risk for bladder cancer. One large case series of 1584 consecutive women undergoing office cystourethroscopy in a single urogynecology center found that the rate of bladder cancer was 1.7% in women with microscopic hematuria. Moreover, most cases of bladder cancer presented with normal initial dipstick urinalysis,[8] which would suggest that persistent symptoms alone may be sufficient to support a diagnostic cystourethroscopy. The author uses a combination of risk factors and objective findings to direct the use of diagnostic cystourethroscopy.

Summary

Cystourethroscopy is feasible, has low morbidity, and should be used conservatively in an FPMRS practice.

PROCEDURES FOR STRESS URINARY INCONTINENCE

Single-Incision Slings

Single-incision mini-slings were introduced as a less invasive surgical option than traditional sling and retropubic urethropexy procedures for stress urinary incontinence. There have been reports of the placement of single-incision slings in the office setting.[9,10] However, many of these data were presented for a sling that is no longer on the market. The role of these procedures in the management of stress urinary incontinence remains controversial, because meta-analysis of effectiveness and complications has demonstrated inferiority to traditional retropubic and transobturator midurethral sling procedures.[11] For this reason, these procedures are not described in detail here.

Periurethral Bulking Agents

Periurethral bulking of the proximal urethra has been an accepted treatment for urinary incontinence for many years. Traditionally this procedure is performed in patients who have stress urinary incontinence with very low leak point pressures (<60 mm H_2O) and without urethral hypermobility (**Table 2**). These women are thought to have a more severe form of stress urinary incontinence, termed intrinsic sphincter deficiency (ISD). There are no accepted criteria for patients who are good candidates for bulking procedures, but generally they have a Q-tip test with a straining value of less than 30° and a leak point pressure of 65 cm H_2O or less. One common scenario in which these agents are used is in women who have recurrent stress urinary incontinence after a prior midurethral sling who demonstrate no urethral hypermobility. Efficacy for primary stress urinary incontinence is lower than that for midurethral sling procedures and the Burch procedure, but low morbidity and good accessibility as an office procedure have maintained the role of periurethral bulking in the treatment of stress urinary incontinence.

Technique/procedure

There are multiple agents available for periurethral bulking (**Table 3**). No clinical trials have been performed to demonstrate superiority of any of the agents. There are 2 common techniques for injection of bulking agents.

1. Transurethral urethroscopy is performed using a rigid cystoscope with a telescope from 0° to 30° and a 20F sheath. The bridge must contain an operating channel that will accommodate the injection needle. Some products offer a built-in needle-delivery system. The patient should be prepared with disinfectant, and xylocaine gel and/or injection of 1% lidocaine around the urethra. The cystoscope is inserted into the bladder and then withdrawn to visualize the proximal urethra. The goal is to inject the bulking material into the superficial muscle (the internal urethral sphincter) at the level of the proximal urethra. Typically the needle is inserted into the mucosa of the urethra, 2 cm distal to the bladder neck, and is advanced 1 cm in the submucosa where the injection is then performed. Injection sites vary by physician preference. The author injects at the 4 o'clock and 8 o'clock positions. All of the agents recommend that once the initial injection is performed, the operator maintain the needle in its position for some time (30 seconds) after the bulking agent is injected to reduce spillage of the material. The volume injected varies by product.
2. In the periurethral method, 1 mL of 1% lidocaine is injected by entering the periurethral tissue at the level of the Skene ducts bilaterally. The urethroscope is then

Table 2
Indications and contraindications to periurethral bulking procedures

Possible Indications	Contraindications
Recurrent stress urinary incontinence after prior sling procedure with no urethral hypermobility	None
The very elderly patient with multiple comorbidities who cannot undergo anesthesia	
Patient with recurrent incontinence after removal of a sling because of complications, who refuses repeat sling of any type and refuses abdominal surgery	

Table 3
Available periurethral bulking agents approved by the US Food and Drug Administration

Product Name	Material
Coaptite (Bioform Medical Inc, San Mateo, CA)	Calcium hydroxylapatite
Durasphere (Carbon Medical Technologies Inc, St Paul, MN)	Pyrolitic carbon-coated zirconium oxide beads
Macroplastique (Uroplasty BV, Geleen, The Netherlands)	Polydimethyl-siloxane macroparticles
Tegress (CR Bard Inc, Covington, GA)	Ethylene vinyl copolymer

inserted and the proximal urethra is visualized. The needle is inserted periurethrally and is advanced submucosally under direct urethroscopic visualization to the proximal urethra, where the bulking agent is injected.

Complications and management

The most common complication is pain during injection, which can be minimized by injection of lidocaine before the procedure. Urinary tract infection occurs in 10% to 15% of cases. The author's practice is to administer perioperative antibiotics for 24 hours. Urinary retention may occur, and is best treated with instructing the patient to perform clean intermittent catheterization, as an indwelling catheter may affect the efficacy of the bulking agent. Finally, suburethral abscess has been reported, which would require antibiotic therapy and, possibly, debridement.

Postoperative care

Patients are given perioperative antibiotic prophylaxis for 24 hours. Pain control can be accomplished with nonsteroidal anti-inflammatory drugs and a warm bath. If the patient develops urinary retention, clean intermittent catheterization (CIC) is taught, and close follow-up is required to avoid unnecessary prolonged CIC, which may influence the effectiveness of the bulking agent.

Reporting, follow-up, and clinical implications

Periurethral bulking is documented as a separate procedure note. Patients should return at 2 weeks to be assessed for efficacy and complications. If patients have not had significant improvement, a repeat injection is scheduled within 4 weeks. If no improvement is seen after the second injection, further injections are unlikely to help.

Outcomes

The quality of the data for periurethral bulking agents is poor. Most of the studies are cohort studies or case series performed in women with uncomplicated stress urinary incontinence, which is not the patient population for which most FPMRS physicians use this therapy. A recent Cochrane review concluded that the current data are insufficient to guide clinical practice,[12] and also commented that the existing trials were small and of moderate quality. Midurethral slings and the Burch procedure are superior to periurethral bulking in uncomplicated primary stress urinary incontinence.

Controversies

Whether periurethral bulking agents work well in patients with stress urinary incontinence with a stable urethra, or in very elderly and ill patients, remains unanswered. However, the lack of other treatment options for this group of patients secures the ongoing role of periurethral bulking agents in the treatment of stress urinary incontinence.

PROCEDURES FOR URGE URINARY INCONTINENCE AND OVERACTIVE BLADDER

Percutaneous Nerve Evaluation

Sacral neuromodulation is increasingly used for refractory idiopathic overactive bladder, urinary retention, fecal incontinence, and pelvic pain syndromes (**Table 4**). Because all patients do not respond to sacral neuromodulation, a trial of the therapy is performed. Testing for efficacy of sacral neuromodulation consists of either a staged outpatient procedure whereby 2 surgeries involves the placement of a quadripolar lead in the operating room, or an initial testing performed in the office setting as a percutaneous nerve evaluation (PNE). PNE is an office technique whereby a monopolar, temporary lead is placed. The nature of fecal incontinence and pelvic pain syndrome may necessitate a longer trial period to determine whether the therapy is effective. Therefore, when a trial of sacral neuromodulation is attempted for a patient with one of these conditions, the trial is generally performed after placement of a permanent lead in the operating room.

Technique/procedure

The patient is placed in the prone position on the examination table and disinfectant is applied. The location of the third sacral foramen is estimated. This estimation consists of measuring 9 cm cephalad from the tip of the coccyx and then measuring 2 cm laterally; this location represents the location of the S3 foramen. The needle insertion site is 2 cm directly cephalad to this point. The selected area is then injected with 1% lidocaine with epinephrine, paying careful attention to avoid injecting within the foramen, which could affect the motor response that the operator is attempting to elicit. The needle is inserted at a sixty degree angle to the skin and is adjusted until it is found to be within the S3 foramen. Confirmation of placement is by observation of the correct sensory response of vibrations in the vagina or rectum, observation of plantarflexion of the ipsilateral great toe, and contraction of the pelvic floor muscles. The obturator within the needle is removed and the temporary lead is inserted. The needle is then withdrawn while the temporary lead is stabilized to minimize migration. Many clinicians insert leads bilaterally during the test phase.

Complications and management

The most common complication during the test phase is lead migration. The temporary lead is not tined and therefore, is prone to moving. Infection is uncommon because the trial phase is short.

Postoperative care

Many physicians advocate for treatment with cephalexin or trimethoprim-sulfamethoxazole during the trial phase. Patients are instructed to keep a bladder diary. If bilateral leads have been inserted, the patient is instructed to switch the external stimulator from one lead to the other, and to do this after 2 days on the first side. The test phase lasts from 4 to 7 days, after which the patient returns to the office for removal of the temporary leads and to determine whether they have had a sufficient response to warrant permanent implantation.

Table 4
Indications and contraindications for percutaneous nerve evaluation

Indications	Contraindications
Refractory idiopathic overactive bladder	Diathermy
Idiopathic urinary retention	—

Reporting, follow-up, and clinical implications
This procedure is documented as a separate procedure note. Patients are followed up in 5 to 7 days for removal of the temporary lead and to discuss implantation. If the patient has an equivocal or negative response, the options are to proceed with implantation of a permanent tined lead under anesthesia, with a subsequent trial period, or move on to other therapies such as intravesical injection of onabotulinumtoxinA.

Outcomes
PNE will elicit a positive clinical response that leads to permanent implantation in 40% to 50% of patients.[13,14]

Controversies
It is clear that staged implantation has a higher rate of implantation of the permanent device in comparison with PNE (70%–90% vs 40%–50%).[13,14] Furthermore, the majority of patients who fail a PNE trial will have a clinical response to a tined-lead implant.[15] However, this study also showed that a nearly 100% implantation rate can be achieved if 4 trials of implantation are performed, suggesting that an α error may be generated if enough tests are performed. There is no difference in the specificity of a positive trial between staged implantation and PNE.[16]

The question of whether there is a role for PNE in clinical practice is an important one. The simplicity and safety of office-based PNE increases the availability of testing for this important therapy to elderly women who may be reluctant to undergo 2 procedures in the operating room. Furthermore, the data supporting staged implantation versus PNE come from small series. Finally, several interests compete in this debate, as physicians have higher total reimbursements for PNE compared with staged implantation, but the hospital and insurance companies may encounter lower costs. Consequently, some insurance companies require PNE evaluation before the more costly implant of the permanent lead.[14] Cost-effectiveness analysis is difficult because the quality of the data is only moderate.

Intravesical Injection of OnabotulinumtoxinA

OnabotulinumtoxinA injection for the treatment of refractory overactive bladder was approved by the Food and Drug Administration in January 2013. OnabotulinumtoxinA was previously approved for hyperreflexic neurogenic bladder. Patients with refractory overactive bladder currently have the treatment options of neuromodulation or intradetrusor onabotulinumtoxinA injection.

Technique/procedure
This technique is as described in the cystoscopy section.

Complications and management
The main additional complication of the injection of onabotulinumtoxinA, beyond the risks of cystoscopy alone, is the risk of urinary retention. Urinary retention requiring catheterization is reported in 5% to 11% of women who receive an injection of 100 units.[3,17] Urinary retention may present 2 to 4 weeks after the procedure and will last an average of 6 to 8 weeks. Patients are instructed on the technique of intermittent self-catheterization. No antibiotic prophylaxis is indicated.

Postoperative care
Urinary tract infection occurs in 33% of patients.[3] The author's practice is to treat with a 3-day course of antibiotics after the injection.

Reporting, follow-up, and clinical implications

This procedure is documented as a separate procedure note. In the author's practice, patients are followed up in 14 days for a postvoid residual volume check and to assess response. Clinical response may improve for up to 4 weeks after the procedure. The injection may be repeated once the clinical efficacy declines. The average time to repeat injection is 6 months. It is generally accepted that the injection should not be repeated within 12 weeks.

Outcomes

Nearly all women will have a clinical response to onabotulinumtoxinA injection (95%). Subjective cure is twice as common with onabotulinumtoxinA injection than with oral anticholinergics (13% vs 27%).[3]

Controversies

The long-term effect of repeated intradetrusor injection of onabotulinumtoxinA has not been established.

Posterior Tibial Nerve Stimulation

Posterior tibial nerve stimulation is another treatment option for refractory overactive bladder. This procedure provides stimulation of the posterior tibial nerve, which carries electric impulses to the sacral nerve plexus, where its mechanism of action is thought to be similar to that of sacral neuromodulation. This procedure is performed entirely in the office setting.

Technique/procedure

The patient is counseled at the beginning of the treatment cycle. Patients undergo 12 consecutive weekly treatments. The patient sits comfortably in a chair with one of her feet elevated. The clinician marks a point that is 3 finger-breadths cephalad to the middle of the ankle, and 1 finger-breadth posterior to the tibia. This location is marked and cleaned with an alcohol swab. The clinician inserts a small needle electrode into the skin, breaking through the dermis quickly by tapping on the electrode. Then a grounding pad is placed along the bottom of the ipsilateral foot, and a stimulator is connected to the needle electrode with a lead wire. The stimulator is then turned on and the stimulus is slowly increased to the point where the patient demonstrates flexion of the great toe, or fanning of the toes. The patient may experience a sensation in the bottom of the foot, the heel, and along the leg. Once this is achieved, the stimulator is left on for 30 minutes. After the therapy is complete, the needle is removed and the patient is instructed to return for the next weekly appointment. Clinical response should be assessed by a bladder diary after the 12th treatment.

Complications and management

The most common side effects are mild pain or skin inflammation at the stimulation site, which can be managed with nonsteroidal anti-inflammatory agents.

Postoperative care

Patients may immediately resume their normal activities.

Reporting, follow-up, and clinical implications

Procedure notes should be documented. There is no standard for following patients over the longer term once the therapy is complete. Common practice is to repeat an abbreviated course of therapy if overactive bladder symptoms return.

Outcomes

Long-term efficacy and outcomes remain unknown. However, clinical trials have shown good short-term results, with response rates reported from 54% to 94%.[18,19]

Controversies

The main controversy surrounding the use of posterior tibial nerve stimulation is the continued lack of long-term data.

PROCEDURES TO CORRECT SURGICAL COMPLICATIONS

Mesh Exposure

The use of synthetic polypropylene mesh in the treatment of pelvic floor disorders is increasing, despite some concerns regarding complications of pain and mesh exposure. The rate of mesh-related complications with transvaginal mesh procedures is 10% for pelvic organ prolapse, 6% for abdominal sacral colpopexy, and 1% to 2% for midurethral sling procedures.[20–22] Most patients with vaginal mesh exposure will present complaining that they feel something within the vagina or that their partner experiences pain during intercourse. Some patients with mesh exposure also complain of pain themselves. The most appropriate initial treatment for small mesh exposure (<0.5 cm) is treatment with topical estrogen. If the exposure persists, resection of the visible mesh should be performed. This procedure can often be accomplished in the office setting.[23]

Technique/procedure

The patient should be counseled, and the erosion site cleaned with disinfectant. The exposed mesh should be trimmed down to the level of the vaginal epithelium using scissors. Some clinicians advocate injecting first with 1% lidocaine and trimming to just below the surface of the epithelium until a bleeding edge is encountered. There is no evidence regarding the optimal way to perform this procedure.[24]

Complications and management

The most common complication is pain during the procedure, although this procedure is generally well tolerated. The surgeon should not be reluctant to use local anesthesia liberally. Infection is rare, and prophylactic antibiotics are not indicated. Recurrent mesh exposure may be managed with a second outpatient trimming, or with examination under anesthesia and removal in the operating room.

Postoperative care

Patients are instructed to treat with 0.5 to 1 g of transvaginal estrogen cream (conjugated estrogen or estradiol) daily for 4 weeks. The author does not routinely treat with antibiotics. Repeat trimming may be indicated, and the decision of whether to repeat the trimming in the office or to proceed to the operating room should be discussed with the patient.

Reporting, follow-up, and clinical implications

This procedure is documented as a separate procedure note. Patients are seen in the clinic within 2 weeks to assess for progress.

Outcomes

Small areas of vaginal mesh exposure can be managed successfully in the office setting for most patients.

Controversies

Several risk factors have been identified in vaginal exposure of mesh after incontinence and prolapse procedures that involve mesh. Risk factors include increasing age, smoking, and concomitant hysterectomy with sacral colpopexy. Clinicians should screen these patients more carefully for mesh exposures after pelvic reconstructive surgery.

Sling Adjustment and Release

The midurethral sling (MUS) is the current gold-standard treatment for stress urinary incontinence. One of the complications with MUS procedures is urinary retention (1%–2%).[22,25] Risk factors for urinary retention include young age, concomitant anterior or apical prolapse procedure, and stage 3 or 4 vaginal apical descent.[25,26] Reliable predictors of urinary retention have not been identified. The options for treating postoperative urinary retention include sling adjustment and sling release. Sling adjustment involves loosening the sling by pulling down with an instrument within the urethra, or opening the vaginal incision and placing an instrument between the urethra and the sling. Sling release involves opening the vaginal incision and dividing the sling in the midline. Sling adjustment and sling release have been described in the office setting.

Sling-adjustment procedures are generally performed within 10 to 14 days of the sling surgery, because tissue ingrowth will not allow for adjustment beyond that time period. Sling release is performed 2 to 6 weeks following the procedure. There are very limited data available to guide decision making regarding the management of urinary retention after midurethral sling procedures.[25,27]

Technique/procedure

The patient is counseled and the area is cleaned with disinfectant. The vaginal epithelium around the incision site is injected with 5 mL of 1% lidocaine with epinephrine. After 5 minutes, the suture is divided and the vaginal epithelium is separated along the sling incision. The sling should be immediately visible behind the vaginal epithelium, and Metzenbaum scissors can be placed between the sling and the urethra to free the sling in order to completely divide it. The scissors are then used to divide the sling in the midline. Depending on the severity of the retention, the physician may choose to perform very limited urethrolysis by freeing the sling laterally on both sides. The area is then irrigated with normal saline, and the vaginal epithelium is reapproximated using 3-0 Vicryl sutures in a running fashion.

Complications and management

There are no robust data on the frequency of complications from this procedure. Complications may include bleeding, infection, and ongoing urinary retention. Bleeding can be managed with vaginal packing.

Postoperative care

After the procedure is concluded and the patient has recovered sufficiently to ambulate, a voiding trial may be performed to assess for voiding dysfunction. Use of antibiotics is at the discretion of the surgeon. Pretreatment with a fluoroquinolone and continuing for 24 hours is reasonable.

Reporting, follow-up, and clinical implications

The procedure is documented as a separate procedure note. The patient should be seen within 2 weeks to determine whether urinary retention has resolved. If the retention has not resolved, more extensive sling lysis and urethrolysis should be performed in the operating room.

Outcomes

In one small series, immediate resolution of urinary retention was observed in 6 of 7 (86%) patients who underwent in-office sling release.[23]

Controversies

Data supporting this technique are limited to very small case series.

SUMMARY

FPMRS is a growing specialty that is rapidly evolving. Common outpatient procedures within this specialty include cystourethroscopy, procedures for stress and urge urinary incontinence, and procedures to manage postoperative complications.

REFERENCES

1. Denholm SW, Conn IG, Newsam JE, et al. Morbidity following cystoscopy: comparison of flexible and rigid techniques. Br J Urol 1990;66(2):152–4.
2. Chitale S, Hirani M, Swift L, et al. Prospective randomized crossover trial of lubricant gel against an anaesthetic gel for outpatient cystoscopy. Scand J Urol Nephrol 2008;42:164–7.
3. Visco A, Brubaker L, Richter H, et al. Anticholinergic therapy versus onabotulinumtoxinA for urgency urinary incontinence. N Engl J Med 2012;367:1803–13.
4. Garcia-Perdomo HA, Lopez H, Carbonell J, et al. Efficacy of antibiotic prophylaxis in patients undergoing cystoscopy: a randomized clinical trial. World J Urol 2013. [Epub ahead of print].
5. Turan H, Balci U, Erdinc FS, et al. Bacteriuria, pyuria and bacteremia frequency following outpatient cystoscopy. Int J Urol 2006;13:25–8.
6. Cundiff GW, McLennan MT, Bent AE. Randomized trial of antibiotic prophylaxis for combined urodynamics and cystourethroscopy. Obstet Gynecol 1999;93: 749–52.
7. Fantl JA, Newman DK, Colling J, et al. Urinary incontinence in adults: acute and chronic management. Clinical Practice Guideline, No. 2, 1996 Update. U.S. Department of Health and Human Services. Public Health Service, Agency for Health Care Policy and Research. Rockville (MD): AHCPR; 1996. Publication No. 96-0682.
8. Goldberg RP, Sherman W, Sand PK. Cystoscopy for lower urinary tract symptoms in urogynecologic practice: the likelihood of finding bladder cancer. Int Urogynecol J Pelvic Floor Dysfunct 2008;19:991–4.
9. Presthus JB, Van Drie D, Graham C. MiniArc single-incision sling in the office setting. J Minim Invasive Gynecol 2012;19(3):331–8.
10. Khandwala S, Jayachandran C. TVT-Secur in office sling procedure under local anesthesia: a prospective 2-year analysis. Female Pelvic Med Reconstr Surg 2012;18:233–8.
11. Abdel-Fattah M, Ford JA, Lim CP, et al. Single-incision mini-slings versus standard midurethral slings in surgical management of female stress urinary incontinence: a met-analysis of effectiveness and complications. Eur Urol 2011;60: 468–80.
12. Kirchin V, Page T, Keegan PE, et al. Urethral injection therapy for urinary incontinence in women. Cochrane Database Syst Rev 2012;2:CD003881.
13. Borawski K, Foster R, Webster G, et al. Predicting implantation with a neuromodulator using two different test stimulation techniques: a prospective randomized study in urge incontinent women. Neurourol Urodyn 2007;26:14–8.
14. Baxter C, Kim JH. Contrasting the percutaneous nerve evaluation versus staged implantation in sacral neuromodulation. Curr Urol Rep 2010;11:310–4.
15. Sutherland SE, Lavers A, Carlson A, et al. Sacral nerve stimulation for voiding dysfunction: one institution's 11-year experience. Neurourol Urodyn 2007;26:19–28.

16. Kessler TM, Madersbacher H, Kiss G. Prolonged sacral neuromodulation testing using permanent leads: a more reliable patient selection method? Eur Urol 2005; 47:660–5.
17. Dmochowski R, Chapple C, Nitti VW, et al. Efficacy and safety of onabotulinumA for idiopathic overactive bladder: a double-blind, placebo controlled, randomized, dose ranging trial. J Urol 2010;184:2416–22.
18. Peters KM, Carrico DJ, Perez-Marrero RA, et al. Randomized trial of percutaneous tibial nerve stimulation versus sham efficacy in the treatment of overactive bladder syndrome: results from the SUmiT Trial. J Urol 2010;183(4):1438–43.
19. Finazzi-Agro E, Petta F, Sciobica F, et al. Percutaneous tibial nerve stimulation effects on detrusor overactivity incontinence are not due to a placebo effect: a randomized, double-blind, placebo controlled trial. J Urol 2010;184(5):2001–6.
20. Abed H, Rahn DD, Lowenstein L, et al. Incidence and management of graft erosion, wound granulation, and dyspareunia following vaginal prolapse repair with graft materials: a systematic review. Int Urogynecol J 2011;22:789–98.
21. Cundiff GW, Varner E, Visco AG, et al. Risk factors for mesh/suture erosion following sacral colpopexy. Am J Obstet Gynecol 2008;199:688.
22. Richter HE, Albo ME, Zyczynski HM, et al. Retropubic versus transobturator midurethral slings for stress incontinence. N Engl J Med 2010;362:2066–76.
23. Greiman A, Kielb S. Revisions of midurethral slings can be accomplished in the office. J Urol 2012;188:190–3.
24. Davila GW, Jijon A. Managing vaginal mesh exposure/erosions. Curr Opin Obstet Gynecol 2012;24:343–8.
25. Jonsson Funk M, Siddiqui NY, Pate V, et al. Sling revision/removal for mesh erosion and urinary retention: long-term risk and predictors. Am J Obstet Gynecol 2013;208:73.e1–7.
26. Komesu YM, Rogers RG, Kammerer-Doak DN, et al. Clinical predictors of urinary retention after pelvic reconstructive and stress urinary incontinence surgery. J Reprod Med 2007;52:611–5.
27. Hashim H, Terry TR. Management of recurrent stress urinary incontinence and urinary retention following midurethral sling insertion in women. Ann R Coll Surg Engl 2012;94:517–22.

Reimbursement for Office-Based Gynecologic Procedures

Jordan Pritzker, MD, MBA, FACOG

KEYWORDS

- Gynecologic procedures • Reimbursement • Office-based • Coding

KEY POINTS

- Physicians and third-party payers are required to use uniform coding systems mandated by federal law.
- The Health Insurance Portability and Accountability Act of 1996 (HIPAA) established the use of the Healthcare Common Procedural Coding System (which includes the *Current Procedural Terminology* [*CPT*] code set) and the *International Classification of Disease, Ninth Revision, Clinical Modification* (the *ICD-9-CM* code set).
- Reimbursement for office-based gynecologic procedures requires correct coding of what (the procedure) was performed (the CPT code) and why (the diagnosis) it was performed (the *ICD* code).

Reimbursement for office-based gynecologic procedures varies with the contractual obligations that the physician has with the payers involved with the care of a particular patient. The payers may be patients without health insurance coverage (self-pay) or patients with third-party health insurance coverage, such as an employer-based commercial insurance carrier or a government program (eg, Medicare [federal] or Medicaid [state-based]). This article discusses the reimbursement for office-based gynecologic procedures by third-party payers.

Physicians and third-party payers are required to use uniform coding systems mandated by federal law. The Health Insurance Portability and Accountability Act of 1996 (HIPAA) established the use of the Healthcare Common Procedural Coding System (HCPCS) (which includes the *Current Procedural Terminology* [*CPT*] code set) and the *International Classification of Disease, Ninth Revision, Clinical Modification* (the *ICD-9-CM* code set). In October 2003, the HIPAA initiated requirements for most physicians to submit claims electronically to Medicare. On January 1, 2012, the 5010 HIPAA transaction standard was implemented in preparation for the conversion to the *International Classification of Disease, Tenth Revision, Clinical Modification* (*ICD-10-CM*) on October 1, 2014. Most commercial third-party payers prefer electronic submission of claims and, oftentimes, reimburse faster on an electronically submitted clean claim.

Women's Health & Wellness, 155 Froehlich Farm Boulevard, Woodbury, NY 11797, USA
E-mail address: jgpritzker@aol.com

Obstet Gynecol Clin N Am 40 (2013) 787–795
http://dx.doi.org/10.1016/j.ogc.2013.09.002 **obgyn.theclinics.com**
0889-8545/13/$ – see front matter

HCPCS codes were developed by the Centers for Medicare and Medicaid Services (CMS) in 1983 to report services and supplies provided to the government's Medicare and Medicaid programs. The HCPCS is divided into level I and level II codes. Level I codes are those found in the *CPT* book. These codes include category 1, 2, and 3 codes and are updated annually by the American Medical Association (AMA) *CPT* Editorial Panel. Category 1 codes are 5-digit codes used to describe the cognitive, procedural, and material services provided by a physician. Category 2 codes are 4-digits followed by a letter *F*. F codes are tracking codes used to facilitate the collection of information about the quality of care using nationally established performance measures. Category 3 codes are 4-digit codes followed by a letter *T*. T codes are temporary tracking codes that allow the collection of a specific date to assess the clinical efficacy, use, and outcomes of emerging technologies. Level II HCPCS codes are temporary and permanent codes used to report services that are not covered by *CPT* codes. These codes include codes for supplies, durable medical equipment, the National Drug Codes (NDC) J-codes for drugs given by a method other than oral administration, and the temporary G and Q codes. The CMS HCPCS Workgroup updates these codes.

The *ICD-9-CM* is the diagnosis code set that has been used for submission of claims to third-party payers in the United States. The *ICD-10-CM* was developed by the World Health Organization in 1994 and is currently used in many countries throughout the world. As of October 1, 2014, providers and payers in the United States are required to use the *ICD-10-CM* for payment. The *ICD-10-CM* diagnosis codes have 3 to 7 digits and begin with a letter. There are 21 chapters of the 68 000 codes in this code set. Obstetric conditions begin with the letter *O*. This code set is intended to enable increased specificity in reporting diseases and conditions, including primary care encounters, external causes of injury, mental disorders, neoplasms, preventive health, socioeconomic details, ambulatory care conditions, lifestyle problems, and screening tests. *ICD–9–CM* to *ICD-10* crosswalk tables have been developed.

Reimbursement for office-based gynecologic procedures requires correct coding of what (the procedure) was performed (the *CPT* code) and why (the diagnosis) it was performed (the *ICD* code). For a third party payer to reimburse for a service or procedure, the service or procedure and diagnosis must be a covered benefit and medically necessary in accordance with the patient's health insurance benefit's contract. Payers may request clinical records and operative reports before adjudicating a claim for payment. The documentation in the clinical record must support the indications for the procedure performed and the operative report must support the procedure of record on the claim submitted to the payer. Of course, the documentation of hand written records must be legible for validation of indication and procedure performed. Reimbursement for multiple procedures on the same date of service may be subject to NCCI edits (National Correct Coding Initiative Edits as proposed by a third-party entity for CMS) and individual payer surgical bundling rules, including modifier rules and sequencing of procedure rules. The *ICD* diagnosis codes should be to the highest degree of specificity and the highest degree of certainty for the procedure being performed. The *ICD* diagnosis should be relevant and linked to the applicable *CPT* procedure code on the claim. The *ICD* diagnosis codes should be sequenced in order of relevance to the associated procedure on the claim.

GLOBAL SURGICAL PACKAGE

The *CPT* codes are based on a global surgical package for the particular procedure. The global surgical package includes all of the necessary services normally provided by the surgeon before, during, and after the procedure. Most payers consider surgeons in the same specialty and in the same group as a single provider. The AMA *CPT* global surgical package varies slightly from the Medicare global surgical package. In 1992, a uniform definition of the Medicare global surgical package was published with the implementation of the Medicare Physician Fee Schedule based on the Resource-Based Relative Value Scale. The AMA/Specialty Society Relative Value System Update Committee provides recommendations to the CMS of the work relative value units (RVUs) and the practice expense component of the *CPT* codes. The Medicare global surgical package includes a description of preoperative services, intraoperative services, and postoperative services. The postoperative services for many procedures include a global surgical period (0, 10, or 90 days) of related care based on the procedure performed. Office-based gynecologic procedures are generally considered minor procedures by Medicare and usually have a 0- or 10-day global surgical period. Ten-day global surgical periods include all services provided pertaining to the procedure for 10 days after the procedure and usually include one postoperative office visit with the payment for the procedure. Most payers follow the global surgical package as published by the CMS.

The following services are included in the *CPT* global surgery package:

- The operation
- Local infiltration
- One related evaluation and management (E&M) encounter on the date immediately before or on the same date of the procedure (including history and physical examination)
- Written orders
- Evaluation of patients in the postanesthesia recovery unit
- Immediate postoperative care, including dictating operative notes and talking with the family and other physicians
- Typical postoperative follow-up care
- Supplies and materials usually included in the procedure

The preservice work includes the following:

- Paperwork from hospital admission, including interval history and physical examination, record review
- Obtain operative consent
- Check instrumentation and materials
- Position and drape patients after anesthesia induction
- Scrub, gown, and glove

The intraservice work includes the procedure from skin incision to skin closure, if performed, or from the placement of instrumentation to the removal of primary surgical instrumentation.

The postservice work includes the following:

- Accompany patients to the recovery room and observe until stable
- Write orders
- Speak with family
- Dictate operative report
- Postprocedure visits within the global surgical period as applicable

E&M SERVICES

The office encounter for the evaluation of patients for the office-based gynecologic procedure may be reimbursable. This reimbursement is based both on *CPT* rules for new patients or established patients as well as on the fulfillment of the levels of the 3 key components of the *CPT* code: history, physical examination, and medical decision making (MDM).

SURGICAL MODIFIERS

Surgical modifiers indicate that a service has been modified or that additional services have been provided that are not included in the procedure performed. Modifiers that may be applicable to the office-based gynecologic procedures include the following:

Modifier 25: Significant, separately identifiable E&M service provided by the same physician on the same day of the procedure or other service
Modifier 52: Reduced services
Modifier 53: Discontinued Procedure
Modifier 57: Decision for surgery

Modifier 25 is applied to an E&M code if a separately identifiable E&M service has been provided that is substantiated by the documentation and is unrelated to the procedure performed. Modifier 52 is applied to the *CPT* code if the procedure is reduced at the physician's discretion or if all portions of the procedure could not be completed. Payment for these modifiers may vary by payer rules. Modifier 53 is appended to the procedure code if the procedure could not be performed because of extenuating circumstances or the well-being of patients. Modifier 57 is appended to the E&M code if the visit results in the procedure being performed on the same date of service.

FACILITY FEES FOR OFFICE-BASED SURGERY

The value of the *CPT* code for office-based gynecologic procedures includes a practice expense component in the *CPT* code payment. This payment is demonstrated in the difference in values for the *facility* RVU versus the *nonfacility* RVU for a *CPT* code. For example, the RVUs for the facility for *CPT* code 58555 (hysteroscopy, diagnostic [separate procedure]) is 5.67, and the *nonfacility* RVUs are 8.56. The latter includes reimbursement for the practice expenses incurred by performing the procedure in the office setting as opposed to the physician performing the procedure in the hospital or in an ambulatory surgery center. A similar example is for the hysteroscopic tubal sterilization procedures (*CPT* code 58565). The RVUs for the *facility* for *CPT* code 58565 is 13.02 and the *nonfacility* RVUs is 57.73. The latter includes reimbursement for the practice expenses incurred by performing the procedure in the office setting as well as the tubal insert devices.

Many payers will not reimburse a facility fee for office-based procedures unless the office is properly licensed by the state where the facility operates. Specifically, the facility must be licensed as an ambulatory surgical center or a comparable title used by a state's licensing law to describe a freestanding facility, other than a physician's office, where surgical and diagnostic services are provided on an ambulatory basis.

Reimbursement for Pain Relief of Office-Based Gynecologic Procedures

Most office-based gynecologic procedures do not require the administration of anesthesia. For those office-based procedures that typically use local anesthesia, the practice expense portion of the RVUs of the *CPT* codes of the office-based procedure includes the costs of the resources for the provision of the anesthetic.

By various state laws, office-based procedures differ from office-based surgery in that the latter is defined as any surgical or other invasive procedure performed by a physician, physician assistant, or specialist assistant, outside of a hospital, diagnostic and treatment center, ambulatory surgery center, or other Public Health Law Article 28 facility in which moderate or deep sedation or general anesthesia is used. In general, gynecologic procedures that are being performed in the office-based setting do not require sedation or general anesthesia.

Only 2 gynecologic procedure codes have conscious sedation included in the codes. These codes are 57155 (insertion of uterine tandem and/or vaginal ovoids for clinical brachytherapy) and 58823 (drainage of pelvic abscess, transvaginal or transrectal approach, percutaneous) and are usually not performed in the office setting.

Reimbursement for Surgical Abortion in the Office Setting

CPT codes
- 59812 Treatment of incomplete abortion, any trimester, completed surgically
- 59820 Treatment of missed abortion, completed surgically, first trimester
- 59830 Treatment of septic abortion, completed surgically
- 59840 Induced abortion, by dilation and curettage
- 59841 Induced abortion, by dilation and evacuation

Common *ICD-9-CM* codes
- 632 Missed abortion
- 634.X1 Incomplete abortion
- 635.XX Legally induced abortion (*X* indicates fourth and fifth digit required as indicated)

Office-based surgical interruption of pregnancy, depending on the provider experience and resources, may be performed through the first trimester (up to 13 weeks, 6 days' gestation). Injection of local anesthesia, when administered, is included in the *CPT* procedure code and not billable separately from the procedure. However, a paracervical block (*CPT* 64435) may or may not be billable depending on the payment policies of the payer.

Reimbursement for Hysteroscopy and Hysteroscopic Sterilization in the Office Setting

CPT codes
- 58555 Hysteroscopy, diagnostic (separate procedure)
- 58558 Hysteroscopy, surgical; with sampling (biopsy) of endometrium and/or polypectomy, with or without dilation and curettage
- 58565 Hysteroscopy, surgical, with bilateral fallopian tube cannulation to induce occlusion by placement of permanent implants

Common *ICD-9-CM* codes
- 621.0 Polyp of corpus uteri
- 626.X Disorders of menstruation
- Other codes as applicable
- V25.2 Sterilization, admission for interruption of fallopian tubes or vas deferens (*X* indicates fourth and fifth digit required as indicated)

Diagnostic hysteroscopy (*CPT* code 58555) is a bundled service in *CPT* codes 58558 and 58565 and cannot be reported separately.

There is a product currently available in the United States for performing hysteroscopic sterilization. This product is the Essure Microinsert System. The cost of the permanent implantable contraceptive intratubal occlusion devices and delivery system (HCPCs code A42641) is included in the practice expense of the hysteroscopic sterilization *CPT* code for the nonfacility (office) site of service. For hysteroscopic tubal sterilization procedures (*CPT* code 58565), the RVUs for the facility is 13.02 and the nonfacility RVUs is 57.73. The latter includes reimbursement for the practice expenses incurred by performing the procedure in the office setting as well as the tubal insert devices.

The diagnostic and surgical hysteroscopy codes (58555 and 58558, respectively) have 0-day Medicare global periods, and postprocedure office visits are billable at the appropriate E&M level of care. Hysteroscopic tubal sterilization (*CPT* code 58565) has a 90-day Medicare global period, and the procedure code includes typical postprocedural office visits. The hysterosalpingography that is performed after the procedure to ascertain closure of the fallopian tubes is separately billable when the service occurs.

Modifier 52 should be appended to the procedure code if the permanent implant is placed in only one fallopian tube. This may or may not impact reimbursement depending on the payer policy.

Reimbursement for Global Ablation Techniques

CPT codes
- 58353 Endometrial ablation, thermal, without hysteroscopic guidance
- 58356 Endometrial cryoablation with ultrasonic guidance, including endometrial curettage, when performed
- 58563 Hysteroscopy, surgical, with endometrial ablation (eg, endometrial resection, electrosurgical ablation, thermoablation)

Common *ICD-9-CM* codes
- 621.0 Polyp of corpus uteri
- 626.X Disorders of menstruation

The 3 procedures for global endometrial ablation include the thermal endometrial ablation without hysteroscopic guidance, the endometrial cryoablation with ultrasound guidance procedure, and hysteroscopy with endometrial ablation by resection or thermoablation. The administration of local and paracervical block anesthesia is included in the procedure codes. Procedure codes 58353 and 58356 are 10-day Medicare global day periods and include a postprocedure visit, generally within 2 weeks of the procedure. Procedure code 58563 is a 0-day Medicare global day period; therefore, subsequent office visits after the procedure may be billed at the appropriate level of E&M service provided.

Reimbursement for Intrauterine Device Placement/Removal, Etonogestrel/Nexplanon

CPT Codes
- 11981 Insertion, nonbiodegradable drug-delivery implant
- 11982 Removal, nonbiodegradable drug-delivery implant
- 11983 Removal with reinsertion, nonbiodegradable drug-delivery implant
- 58300 Insertion of intrauterine device (IUD)
- 58301 Removal of IUD

Common *ICD-9-CM* codes
- V25.02 General counseling and advice, initiation of other contraceptives
- V25.1 Insertion of intrauterine contraceptive device
- V25.11 Encounter for insertion of intrauterine contraception
- V25.12 Encounter for removal of intrauterine contraception
- V25.13 Encounter for removal and reinsertion of intrauterine contraception
- V25.5 Insertion of implantable subdermal contraception

The counseling for contraceptive management session may be submitted to the payer if this occurs independent of a preventive/annual examination, which may or may not include a review of patients' history and a physical examination. Therefore, this encounter may be based on time if more than 50% of the visit is spent counseling (MDM) patients. Accordingly, *CPT* E&M (99201–99215) codes may be indicated based on time. For example, if the patient encounter was 30 minutes, with 20 minutes spent counseling an established patient, then 99213 would be assigned. If the nonbiological drug-delivery implant or the IUD was placed on the same day as the counseling session, then add modifier 25 to the E&M service. If a nonbiological drug-delivery implant is removed and replaced on the same date of service, then *CPT* code 11983 is submitted. In the event of the IUD, if patients have an IUD removed and a new one inserted during the same visit, then both the IUD removal (58301) and insertion (58300) are reported. If the IUD insertion could not be performed, modifier 53 is appended to the procedure code 58300.

The cost of the nonbiodegradable drug-delivery implant or IUD is not included in these codes and should be reported separately. The nonbiodegradable drug-delivery implant that is currently marketed in the United States is the etonogestrel contraceptive implant system, which is billed with HCPCS code J7307. The common IUDs used in the United States are the copper IUD and the progesterone IUD. Use HCPCS code J7300 for billing for the copper IUD and HCPCS code J7302 for billing for the progesterone IUD.

Reimbursement for Colposcopy/LEEP/Cryotherapy

CPT codes

- 57420 Colposcopy of the entire vagina, with cervix if present
- 57421 Colposcopy of the entire vagina, with cervix if present, with biopsy of vagina/cervix
- 57452 Colposcopy of the cervix including upper/adjacent vagina
- 57454 Colposcopy with biopsy of the cervix and endocervical curettage
- 57455 Colposcopy with biopsy of the cervix
- 57456 Colposcopy with endocervical curettage
- 57460 Colposcopy with loop electrode biopsy of the cervix
- 57461 Colposcopy with loop electrode conization of the cervix (do not report 57461 in addition to 57456)
- 57510 Cautery of cervix, electrocautery or thermal
- 57511 Cautery of cervix, cryotherapy, initial or repeat
- 57513 Cautery of cervix laser ablation
- 57520 Conization of cervix, with or without fulguration, with or without dilation and curettage, with or without repair; cold knife or laser
- 57522 Conization of cervix, loop electrode excision

Common *ICD-9-CM* codes

- 622.10 Dysplasia of cervix, unspecified
- 622.11 Mild dysplasia of cervix, cervical intraepithelial neoplasia (CIN) I
- 622.12 Moderate dysplasia of cervix, CIN II
- 623.0 Dysplasia of cervix
- 233.1 CIN III, glandular CIN III
- 795.0X Abnormal Papanicolaou smear of cervix and cervical human papillomavirus (HPV)
- 795.1X Abnormal Papanicolaou smear of vagina and vaginal HPV (*X* indicates fifth digit required as indicated)

Cervical colposcopy and procedures specific to the cervix are usually performed in the office setting. The administration of anesthesia, if performed, is included in the valuation of the *CPT* procedure code and not separately billable. *CPT* codes 57420 to 57461 have 0-day Medicare global periods. Therefore, office visits after the procedure are not included in the procedure code and are billable at the appropriate level of E&M service rendered. *CPT* codes 57510 and 57513 have a 10-day Medicare global period and include one postprocedure office visit in the few weeks after the procedure.

Reimbursement for Vulvar Procedures: Biopsy, Treatment of Bartholin Abscess, Treatment of Condyloma

CPT codes

- 56405 Incision and drainage of vulva or perineal abscess
- 56420 Incision and drainage of Bartholin gland abscess
- 56440 Marsupialization of Bartholin gland cyst
- 56441 Lysis of labial adhesions
- 56442 Hymenotomy, simple incision
- 56501 Destruction of lesions, vulva; simple (eg, laser surgery, electrosurgery, cryosurgery, chemosurgery)
- 56505 Biopsy of vulva or perineum (separate procedure), 1 lesion
- +56506 each additional lesion
- 56700 Partial hymenectomy or revision of hymenal ring
- 56820 Colposcopy of vulva
- 56821 Colposcopy of vulva with biopsy
- 57023 Incision and drainage of vaginal hematoma, nonobstetrical (eg, post-trauma, spontaneous bleeding)

Common *ICD-9-CM* codes

- 078.11 Condylomata acuminata
- 616.2 Bartholin duct cyst
- 616.3 Bartholin duct abscess
- 616.4 Other abscess of the vulva
- 624.01 Vulvar intraepithelial neoplasia (VIN I)
- 624.02 VIN II
- 624.03 VIN III
- 624.09 Leukoplakia of vulva
- 624.3 Hypertrophy of vulva
- 624.5 Vulvar hematoma (nonobstetrical)
- 624.6 Polyp of labia and vulva
- 701.0 Lichen sclerosis et atrophicus
- 752.42 Imperforate hymen

The vulvar procedures performed in the office setting include the administration of anesthesia. Separately identifiable E&M services that are provided, substantiated by the documentation, and are unrelated to the procedure performed may be billed with modifier 25 appended to the appropriate E&M service provided.

Vulvar procedures are 0-day Medicare global surgical days, and subsequent office visits are billable at the appropriate level of E&M service provided.

Reimbursement for Cystoscopy and Other Urogynecologic Procedures

CPT codes

- 51726 Complex cystometrogram (ie, calibrated electronic equipment)
- 51727 Complex cystometrogram (ie, calibrated electronic equipment); with urethral pressure profile studies, (ie, urethral closure pressure profile), any technique

51728 Complex cystometrogram (ie, calibrated electronic equipment); with voiding pressure studies (VP) (ie, bladder voiding pressure), any technique
51729 Complex cystometrogram (ie, calibrated electronic equipment); with VP (ie, bladder voiding pressure) and urethral pressure profile studies (ie, urethral closure pressure profile), any technique
51741 Complex uroflowmetry (eg, calibrated electronic equipment)
+51797 VP, intra-abdominal (ie, rectal, gastric, intraperitoneal)
58200 Cystourethroscopy (separate procedure)
52287 Cystourethroscopy, with injections for chemodenervation of the bladder

Common *ICD-9-CM* codes

625.6 Stress incontinence
788.30 Urinary incontinence, unspecified
788.31 Urge incontinence
788.33 Mixed incontinence

Office-based urogynecologic procedures include anesthesia, if administered.

Office-based cystometrics and cystourethroscopy procedures have a 0-day Medicare global period, and subsequent office visits may be billed at the appropriate E&M level of service rendered.

CPT code 51797 is an add-on procedure and is billed with 51728 and 51729, when performed.

When multiple procedures are performed in the same date of service, modifier 51 should be appended to the lower RVU-valued procedure. These procedures performed by, or are under the direct supervision of, a physician or other qualified health care professional and all instruments, equipment, fluids, gases, probes, catheters, technician's fees, medications, gloves, trays, tubing, and other sterile supplies should be provided by that individual and are included in the payment for the *CPT* code. When the provider only interprets the results and/or operates the equipment, a professional component, modifier 26, should be used to identify these services.

REFERENCES

CPT 2013. American Medical Association. AMA 2012. Available at: http://www.ACOG.org/About_ACOG/ACOG_Departments/Coding.

ICD-9-CM Abridged 2011 Diagnostic Coding in Obstetrics and Gynecology. ACOG 2010.

Index

Note: Page numbers of article titles are in **boldface** type.

Obstet Gynecol Clin N Am 40 (2013) 797–805
http://dx.doi.org/10.1016/S0889-8545(13)00106-X

V

W

United States Postal Service

Statement of Ownership, Management, and Circulation
(All Periodicals Publications Except Requestor Publications)

1. Publication Title: Obstetrics and Gynecology Clinics of North America
2. Publication Number: 0 0 0 - 2 7 6
3. Filing Date: 9/14/13
4. Issue Frequency: Mar, Jun, Sep, Dec
5. Number of Issues Published Annually: 4
6. Annual Subscription Price: $293.00
7. Complete Mailing Address of Known Office of Publication (*Not printer*) (*Street, city, county, state, and ZIP+4®*)

Elsevier Inc.
360 Park Avenue South
New York, NY 10010-1710

Contact Person: Stephen R. Bushing
Telephone (Include area code): 215-239-3688

8. Complete Mailing Address of Headquarters or General Business Office of Publisher (*Not printer*)

Elsevier Inc., 360 Park Avenue South, New York, NY 10010-1710

9. Full Names and Complete Mailing Addresses of Publisher, Editor, and Managing Editor (*Do not leave blank*)

Publisher (*Name and complete mailing address*)

Linda Belfus, Elsevier, Inc., 1600 John F. Kennedy Blvd. Suite 1800, Philadelphia, PA 19103-2899

Editor (*Name and complete mailing address*)

Stephanie Donley, Elsevier, Inc., 1600 John F. Kennedy Blvd. Suite 1800, Philadelphia, PA 19103-2899

Managing Editor (*Name and complete mailing address*)

Adrianne Brigido, Elsevier, Inc., 1600 John F. Kennedy Blvd. Suite 1800, Philadelphia, PA 19103-2899

10. Owner (*Do not leave blank. If the publication is owned by a corporation, give the name and address of the corporation immediately followed by the names and addresses of all stockholders owning or holding 1 percent or more of the total amount of stock. If not owned by a corporation, give the names and addresses of the individual owners. If owned by a partnership or other unincorporated firm, give its name and address as well as those of each individual owner. If the publication is published by a nonprofit organization, give its name and address.*)

Full Name	Complete Mailing Address
Wholly owned subsidiary of	1600 John F. Kennedy Blvd., Ste. 1800
Reed/Elsevier, US holdings	Philadelphia, PA 19103-2899

11. Known Bondholders, Mortgagees, and Other Security Holders Owning or Holding 1 Percent or More of Total Amount of Bonds, Mortgages, or Other Securities. If none, check box → ☐ None

Full Name	Complete Mailing Address
N/A	

12. Tax Status (*For completion by nonprofit organizations authorized to mail at nonprofit rates*) (*Check one*)
The purpose, function, and nonprofit status of this organization and the exempt status for federal income tax purposes:
☐ Has Not Changed During Preceding 12 Months
☐ Has Changed During Preceding 12 Months (*Publisher must submit explanation of change with this statement*)

PS Form **3526**, September 2007 (Page 1 of 3 (Instructions Page 3)) PSN 7530-01-000-9931 **PRIVACY NOTICE**: See our Privacy policy in www.usps.com

13. Publication Title: Obstetrics and Gynecology Clinics of North America
14. Issue Date for Circulation Data Below: June 2013

15. Extent and Nature of Circulation			Average No. Copies Each Issue During Preceding 12 Months	No. Copies of Single Issue Published Nearest to Filing Date
a. Total Number of Copies (*Net press run*)			816	743
b. Paid Circulation (By Mail and Outside the Mail)	(1)	Mailed Outside-County Paid Subscriptions Stated on PS Form 3541. (*Include paid distribution above nominal rate, advertiser's proof copies, and exchange copies*)	217	201
	(2)	Mailed In-County Paid Subscriptions Stated on PS Form 3541 (*Include paid distribution above nominal rate, advertiser's proof copies, and exchange copies*)		
	(3)	Paid Distribution Outside the Mails Including Sales Through Dealers and Carriers, Street Vendors, Counter Sales, and Other Paid Distribution Outside USPS®	238	258
	(4)	Paid Distribution by Other Classes Mailed Through the USPS (e.g. First-Class Mail®)		
c. Total Paid Distribution (*Sum of 15b (1), (2), (3), and (4)*) ►			455	459
d. Free or Nominal Rate Distribution (By Mail and Outside the Mail)	(1)	Free or Nominal Rate Outside-County Copies Included on PS Form 3541	55	34
	(2)	Free or Nominal Rate In-County Copies Included on PS Form 3541		
	(3)	Free or Nominal Rate Copies Mailed at Other Classes Through the USPS (e.g. First-Class Mail)		
	(4)	Free or Nominal Rate Distribution Outside the Mail (Carriers or other means)		
e. Total Free or Nominal Rate Distribution (Sum of 15d (1), (2), (3) and (4)			55	34
f. Total Distribution (Sum of 15c and 15e) ►			510	493
g. Copies not Distributed (See instructions to publishers #4 (page #3)) ►			306	250
h. Total (Sum of 15f and g)			816	743
i. Percent Paid (15c divided by 15f times 100) ►			89.22%	93.10%

16. Publication of Statement of Ownership
☐ If the publication is a general publication, publication of this statement is required. Will be printed in the **December 2013** issue of this publication. ☐ Publication not required

17. Signature and Title of Editor, Publisher, Business Manager, or Owner

Stephen R. Bushing –Inventory Distribution Coordinator

Date: September 14, 2013

I certify that all information furnished on this form is true and complete. I understand that anyone who furnishes false or misleading information on this form or who omits material or information requested on the form may be subject to criminal sanctions (including fines and imprisonment) and/or civil sanctions (including civil penalties).

PS Form **3526**, September 2007 (Page 2 of 3)

Moving?

Make sure your subscription moves with you!

To notify us of your new address, find your **Clinics Account Number** (located on your mailing label above your name), and contact customer service at:

Email: journalscustomerservice-usa@elsevier.com

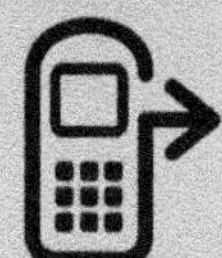

800-654-2452 (subscribers in the U.S. & Canada)
314-447-8871 (subscribers outside of the U.S. & Canada)

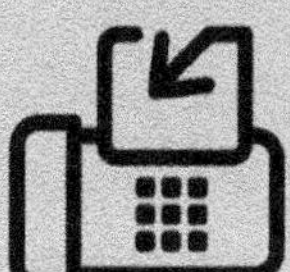

Fax number: 314-447-8029

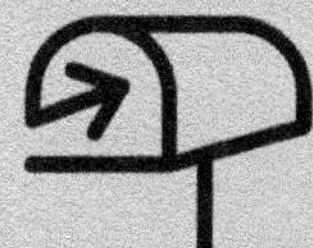

Elsevier Health Sciences Division
Subscription Customer Service
3251 Riverport Lane
Maryland Heights, MO 63043

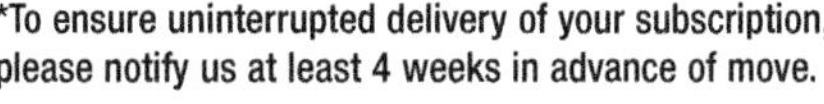

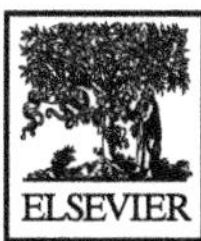

Printed and bound by CPI Group (UK) Ltd, Croydon, CR0 4YY

03/10/2024

01040493-0001